Breakthrough Learning

Quickly Master Applying The Right Material To Be More Fruitful

Donald Mitchell

Author of *Your Breakthroughs,*
2,000 Percent Living, and *Excellent Solutions*
Coauthor of *The 2,000 Percent Solution*

400 Year Project Press
Weston, Massachusetts
United States of America

400 Year Project Books by Donald Mitchell

Your Breakthroughs

Witnessing Made Easy (with Bishop Dale Combs, Lisa Combs, Jim Barbarossa, and Carla Barbarossa)
Ways You Can Witness (with Cherie Hill, Roger de Brabant, Drew Dickens, Gael Torcise, Wendy Lobos, Herpha Jane Obod, and Gisele Umugiraneza)
Investigation Centers

2,000 Percent Living
Help Wanted

The 2,000 Percent Nation

Excellent Solutions (For-Profit and Nonprofit Editions)
Excellent Leadership

The 2,000 Percent Solution (with Carol Coles and Robert Metz)
The Portable 2,000 Percent Solution (with Carol Coles)
The 2,000 Percent Solution Workbook (with Carol Coles)
The 2,000 Percent Squared Solution (with Carol Coles)

The Irresistible Growth Enterprise (with Carol Coles)
The Ultimate Competitive Advantage (with Carol Coles)

Business Basics

Advanced Business
Advanced Business for Innovation
Advanced Business for Social Benefits

Adventures of an Optimist

Breakthrough Learning
Quickly Master Applying the
Right Material to Be More Fruitful

Copyright ©2017 by Donald W. Mitchell
All rights reserved.

No part of this publication may be reproduced, distributed,
or transmitted in any form or by any means,
including photocopying, recording, or other
electronic or mechanical methods without
the prior written permission of the publisher,
except in the case of brief quotations embodied in critical reviews
and certain other noncommercial uses permitted by copyright law.

Scripture taken from the New King James Version®.
Copyright ©1982 by Thomas Nelson, Inc.
Used by permission. All rights reserved.

ISBN: 978-0-692-76041-3
0-692-76041-5

For information, contact:

Donald W. Mitchell
400 Year Project Press
P.O. Box 302
Weston, Massachusetts 02493
781-647-4211

Published in the United States of America

This book is dedicated to:

Breakthrough learners
who apply The 400 Year Project's
and other improvement methods

May quickly and easily learning and applying
Godly lessons always be ahead of them!

And their spouses, their children and grandchildren,
and their descendants

May this book help them to always focus
on the Lord and doing His will!

Contents

Acknowledgments vii
Foreword ix
Introduction xi

Part One: Breakthrough Learning Fundamentals 1

Lesson One: Grasp the Discipline's Approach 5

Lesson Two: Access Relevant Information 15

Lesson Three: Apply Chunks of Information and Knowledge 23

Lesson Four: Update Information and Knowledge 29

Lesson Five: Apply the Discipline 35

Lesson Six: Teach Others and Keep Updating Information
and Knowledge 43

Part Two: Teach Yourself 51

Lesson Seven: Find Descriptions of the Discipline's Approaches 55

Lesson Eight: Determine What Skills Are Required 63

Lesson Nine: Set Goals for Application 69

Lesson Ten: Develop Types and Levels of Skills for Application
in Chunks 77

Lesson Eleven: Learn and Apply an Effective Process in Chunks ... 83

Lesson Twelve: Measure Performance and Have Your
Work Checked 91

Lesson Thirteen: Improve the Process 99

Lesson Fourteen: Update Information and Knowledge —
An Example 107

Lesson Fifteen: Teach Others and Stay Up-to-Date —
An Example 115

Part Three: Teach Others 123

Lesson Sixteen: Assist Learners to Develop Their Goals 131

Lesson Seventeen: Explain the Discipline's Approach and
How to Apply It 137

Lesson Eighteen: Test Learners for Necessary Skills 147

Lesson Nineteen: Demonstrate Multiple Ways to Learn Skills 153

Lesson Twenty: Drill Learners in Skills and Track
Their Progress 161

Lesson Twenty-One: Adjust the Skill-Learning Method 169

Lesson Twenty-Two: Demonstrate Application of the
Discipline to Goals 177

Lesson Twenty-Three: Watch and Correct the
Learner's Application 185

Lesson Twenty-Four: Measure and Address Underlying Causes
of Errors and Slowness 193

Lesson Twenty-Five: Direct the Learner to Self-Improve
the Process 201

Lesson Twenty-Six: Demonstrate How to Update Information
and Knowledge 209

Lesson Twenty-Seven: Improve Your Teaching by Repeating
the Steps for Teaching Others 217

Afterword 225

Appendix A: Donald Mitchell's Testimony 229

Appendix B: Summary of The 400 Year Project 237

Acknowledgments

Oh, give thanks to the LORD!
Call upon His name;
Make known His deeds among the peoples!

— 1 Chronicles 16:8 (NKJV)

I thank Almighty God, our Heavenly Father, for creating the universe and all the people on the Earth; our Lord and Savior, Jesus Christ, for providing the way for us to gain Salvation; and the Holy Spirit for guiding our daily paths towards repentance and righteousness. I also humbly acknowledge the perfect guidance I was sent from God through the Holy Spirit and His Word to write this book. I regret that as an imperfect being I undoubtedly misheard, misunderstood, and misapplied some of that perfect guidance.

I feel deeply honored by Nengarivo Teveli writing the book's excellent foreword. She did outstanding work as my university student concerning ways that education can be improved. I naturally thought of her when it came time to select a foreword author. I was delighted when she kindly agreed to help. I was even more delighted when I saw the foreword, in which she eloquently connects the text of this book to God's command to be fruitful and the Divine potential He has placed in each of us for doing so.

I am grateful to Dr. Peter Drucker for encouraging me to write about 2,000 percent solutions (ways of accomplishing 20 times more with the same or less time, effort, and resources) and to seek ever-simpler ways to help people learn to employ them. His faith in this

Acknowledgments

method for solving problems caused me to take much more seriously the opportunity to share what I had been doing.

I appreciate all those who have permitted me to tell them about 2,000 percent solution methods and the output of The 400 Year Project in improving far beyond these methods. I thank those who have applied what they learned for all the insights I have gained from observing their wonderful work.

I can never thank my family enough for allowing me the time and peace to work on such a huge and awe-inspiring project for God. During the writing, they made many sacrifices without complaining and have been a continual inspiration.

I appreciate my many clients who held off on their demands for my help so that this project could receive the attention it required. Their financial support also made it possible for me to give this time to the Lord and to make this book available.

Finally, I am most appreciative of the many fine improvements that my editor, Bernice Pettinato, made in the text. This is the twenty-first book where she has helped me to make the messages clearer and more pleasant to read. As always, she was a delight to work with. Her kindness made the writing much easier. I value all she has taught me about writing. I'm looking forward to learning new lessons from her during future books.

I accept sole responsibility for any remaining errors and apologize to my readers for any difficulties and inconvenience that they encounter as a consequence.

Foreword

*As iron sharpens iron,
So a man sharpens the countenance of his friend.*

— Proverbs 27:17 (NKJV)

This book is all about sharpening yourself and others in order to use available time, money, efforts, and your other God-given potential to improve all areas of life with exponential results. This is what Professor Donald Mitchell decided to do with all the gifts he has received from God. He has written 21 books on how we human beings can make improvements 20 times faster or accomplish 20 times more than our normal progress.

Ever since I met Professor Mitchell in 2008, when first introduced by Alan Guinn of Rushmore University, I found his books insisting on what God told Adam and Eve in Genesis 1:28 (NKJV), Noah and his sons in Genesis 9:1 (NKJV), Abraham in Genesis 17:6 (NKJV), and Jacob in Genesis 35:11 (NKJV) about being fruitful to be personally motivating. You have the power from God to be similarly fruitful; everyone possesses it. Unfortunately most of us do not know or do not believe that we possess this divine power. In his books, especially in *The 2,000 Percent Solution, 2,000 Percent Living*, and, now, *Breakthrough Learning,* Professor Mitchell reminds us of that power and reveals ways to accomplish this divine purpose of being fruitful. Through describing the methods of The 400 Year Project, he explains how it is possible to achieve astonishing breakthrough results, 20 or more times than you are currently producing, by unlocking your

Foreword

God-given power from the strongholds of fear, stalls, and negative mindsets and beliefs.

In *Breakthrough Learning,* which term Professor Mitchell defines as a method "to learn faster and more effectively," you will learn to quickly master and apply the right material to be more fruitful. The breakthrough learning approaches described in this book enable you to learn and successfully apply what you learn at least 20 times faster and with less time, effort, and resources than others use, even while following what they consider to be the most effective learning and application methods. Professor Mitchell uses a valuable step-by-step method to help you assimilate breakthrough approaches that you can then use to teach others. In doing so, the books embrace what feels like the partial fulfillment of the Apostle Paul's prayer for the Colossians:

> For this reason we also, since the day we heard it, do not cease to pray for you, and to ask that you may be filled with the knowledge of His will in all wisdom and spiritual understanding; that you may walk worthy of the Lord, fully pleasing Him, being fruitful in every good work and increasing in the knowledge of God; strengthened with all might, according to His glorious power, for all patience and longsuffering with joy; giving thanks to the Father who has qualified us to be partakers of the inheritance of the saints in the light. (Colossians 1:9-12, NKJV)

May the integration of the knowledge you learn in *Breakthrough Learning* provide you with a new experience in life and with a reconciled relationship with God's divine power in you. May it empower you to do things faster and more fruitfully, through His Holy Spirit, and become a multiplier of this breakthrough knowledge in your family, church, community, nation, and throughout the world.

Mrs. Nengarivo Teveli
Arusha, Tanzania
July, 2016

Introduction:

Role of Breakthrough Learning

*Let each of us please his neighbor for his good, leading to edification.
For even Christ did not please Himself; but as it is written,
"The reproaches of those who reproached You fell on Me."
For whatever things were written before were written for our learning,
that we through the patience and comfort
of the Scriptures might have hope.
Now may the God of patience and comfort grant you
to be like-minded toward one another, according to Christ Jesus,
that you may with one mind* and *one mouth
glorify the God and Father of our Lord Jesus Christ.*

— Romans 15:2-6 (NKJV)

For accessing and applying truth, people will usually play one of two roles: either as a truth seeker or as a truth teller. As Romans 15:2-6 (NKJV) teaches, no one is going to want to hear the truth from someone who hasn't first developed a pleasing relationship with the potential learner, for which the *truth teller* should be willing to make sacrifices. As a *truth seeker*, however, remember that many of those who know useful truths may be unwilling to sacrifice ... and could even be downright grumpy when approached for help. In such instances, the *truth seeker* may also have to sacrifice to gain their engagement and assistance. Why should truth tellers and seekers be willing to so sacrifice? God directs us to love one another and

Introduction

to serve one another. Seeking, applying, and teaching truth are just three ways of following His commands for loving and serving.

In writing this book, I acknowledge a deep debt to our Heavenly Father; my Lord and Savior, Jesus Christ; and the Holy Spirit. All the eternal truths I know originate from them. I further acknowledge all those who have patiently taught me what I needed to know, keeping at it until I finally saw and acted on the truth.

If anything in this book varies from what the Bible says, please ignore it. Such a divergence is a sign that I have made a mistake. Where that happens, I apologize for having done so and beg your forgiveness.

I also want to point out that I have been taught lessons about breakthrough learning that conflict with some of the effective ways that important truths were taught to me. So keep in mind that this book focuses on *what to do differently to learn what is important in faster, more effective ways*. Part of what to do differently relates to learning on your own, and the other part relates to helping others learn.

I humbly beg your pardon if at any point in this book I seem to be acting without showing sufficient respect to and regard for the many wonderful people who have gone before me in improving and demonstrating better ways to learn. Doing so is not my intention. I merely seek to politely provide breakthrough alternatives, ones that have worked effectively for the people I have taught, as well as for me personally in mastering the knowledge that has provided incalculable benefits to many people through The 400 Year Project (conducted from 1995 through 2015 to develop and demonstrate ways that the whole world can accelerate the rate of improvement in accomplishing its most important tasks, from the mundane to the spiritual, by at least 20 times — see www.fastforward400.com and Appendix B herein).

Why is learning more, faster, and with less effort important? When we ignore an important truth that others know, we can cause disasters for ourselves and others. In other cases, we can miss an important opportunity to benefit. Certainly, whenever we are not learning something we need to know, we are missing valuable opportunities. Whenever we ignore truth, we are also in a poor position to know what would have happened if we had done something differently, especially by doing something more useful.

Some of such truth is ignored because we simply don't realize it exists. Other important truths might be ignored because we don't know how to find them. In some other cases, we see the truth as inconvenient or unpleasant, and choose to set it aside. In still other cases, truth is ignored due to the off-putting manner by which someone has expressed it.

When presented in a pleasing, compelling way, important truths can, instead, delight and lead us to take immediate, helpful actions. When the truth relates to or affects God's Kingdom, quick understanding can be aided by the Holy Spirit, reading the Bible, discussing the matter with other believers, noticing our surroundings, contemplating nature, and praying for enlightenment. Under such ideal directions, few will want to do anything other than take the right action ... as soon as possible.

So what is breakthrough learning? If you believe that Jesus Christ was crucified, died, rose again from the dead, and then ascended into heaven to sit at the right hand of God, and is the Son of our Heavenly Father, and follow Him as your Lord and Savior, then you have already experienced breakthrough learning. Having developed such faith means that the Holy Spirit has entered you and begun to spiritually transform you, causing you to see life more and more from God's perspective and to act accordingly. In God's plan for your life, this experience with breakthrough learning probably wasn't the last one that He intended for you to have.

Let me explain more about what I mean by *breakthrough learning* as described in this book. Like many phrases we meet for the first time, I am sure you have already guessed at what it could mean. Chances are good that one such potential meaning for you is "to learn faster and more effectively." If that's your idea, you are abso-

Introduction

lutely correct. Good for you! If that benefit didn't occur to you, read on anyway. I think you'll like the results of what such learning can bring.

By using the methods described in *Breakthrough Learning*, you should be able to *learn and successfully apply what you learn at least 20 times faster or with 1/21 or less time, effort, and resources than others use, even while following what they consider to be the most effective learning and application methods*. In making this observation, please note that some of the methods described in *2,000 Percent Living* (Salvation Press, 2010) already make available much faster learning and applications of knowledge than what all but a few people usually accomplish. These methods include reading faster with better comprehension, selecting more helpful reading materials, and taking and accessing more useful notes for applying what has been learned. In *Breakthrough Learning*, you will explore still other methods that complement these useful methods to increase your learning effectiveness by at least another increment of 20 times.

What might such a learning experience be like? Where you once would have engaged in most of your important learning alone, you might now seek, instead, the guidance of someone who is a master at such learning to help you quickly identify the simplest elements of what you need to learn, so that you do not have to spend time unnecessarily reviewing what you have already mastered or is unnecessary. As an example, where you might now apply imagination to see other possibilities in solving a problem, such a master might point out that using such imagination in the problem-solving method you are applying can lead to unnecessary errors. Simply appreciating that point might allow you to quickly shift the application of your imagination in ways that would make all the difference. Here's an example. I once observed a history major who was preparing for the Law School Admission Test (LSAT) experience such learning. He read the passages and the logic questions on the test as though he could use any lateral associations that occurred to him to select the correct multiple-choice answers, no matter how little the associations related to the text, rather than narrowly sticking to what the words most clearly indicated. After three hours discussing how to productively narrow the focus of his imagination, this man improved on the LSAT from scoring in the 63rd percentile to reaching the 90th percentile. He had just experienced breakthrough learning.

There's also a second meaning of breakthrough learning: *Make breakthroughs, which are ways of being vastly more effective in applying your own and others' time, money, effort, and other resources to accomplish something important.* One possible way to do so is by learning and effectively applying some of the breakthrough processes developed by The 400 Year Project. These processes include *2,000 percent solutions* (ways of accomplishing 20 times more results with the same or less time, money, and effort), *complementary 2,000 percent solutions* (2,000 percent solutions whose improvements multiply the effectiveness of other 2,000 percent solutions by the same degree), and *excellent solutions* (making one set of changes that have an impact equal to 10 complementary 2,000 percent solutions). The book *2,000 Percent Living* also discusses how to make improvements by using 2,000 percent solutions, as well as with complementary 2,000 percent solutions.

To learn more about these three methods for making breakthroughs, you can find an overview in *Your Breakthroughs* (400 Year Project Press, 2016) by me. Since excellent solutions had not yet been developed when *2,000 Percent Living* was written, this newest and most powerful breakthrough resource needs to be separately studied by you using the for-profit and nonprofit editions of *Excellent Solutions* (400 Year Project Press, 2014) and *Excellent Leadership* (400 Year Project Press, 2015).

What can be accomplished by applying such knowledge? Let me describe the experiences of a student who worked for many years as a shift supervisor in a Middle Eastern fertilizer factory. His most important responsibility was to prepare young Arabs to eventually hold the organization's senior roles. He was effective in such preparation, and all of those with positions above him in the organization

Introduction

were younger men whom he had originally trained. After deciding to earn a doctorate, the student became interested in 2,000 percent solutions. His first 2,000 percent solution project was to study how his factory's profits could be increased by more than 20 times while spending very little money for new investment. He found a way to greatly increase capacity, improve quality, expand productivity, and lower costs that only required an investment equal to about 10 percent of the plant's existing capital base. As a result of making that investment, cash flow expanded by more than 20 times.

Realizing that opportunities to advance his career were constrained in the Middle East, the student moved back to his native country and took a position there with a global producer of basic commodities. As the subject of his Ph.D. dissertation, this man investigated how to create a new business model for his employer, the first major business-model improvement for that industry in more than fifty years. As a result, he discovered a way to lower total costs by over 40 percent, to reduce capital needs by even more, and to expand his company's business volume by several hundred percent. The new business model was approved and pursued by his employer.

Not satisfied with what he had learned and accomplished during the process of attaining his first doctorate, this dedicated learner decided to study for a second one. This time his dissertation work was based on an even more fundamental problem: How to lift poor, uneducated people out of despair and to make their lives hopeful and economically successful. Choosing to serve the village where he grew up, he faithfully trekked hundreds of miles on weekends to teach the people there about 2,000 percent solutions.

Also supported by other volunteers who had once lived there, an initial 50 villagers soon reformed the bad thinking habits that had held them back, began using better thinking processes, formed a cooperative, and began designing and implementing profitable 2,000 percent solutions. In just a few months, most of those 50 people increased their incomes by more than 20 times, reduced their debts by more than 96 percent, slashed the interest rates they were paying on the remaining debt by 96 percent, and increased their net worths by more than 20 times. They also gained new, positive outlooks on life and sought to cooperate with one another rather than be guided by social class distinctions.

What are the key ideas in Breakthrough Learning? A good Broadway musical begins with an overture that gives an entertaining sense of the show. The opening scene grabs our attention and makes us interested in the characters and in finding out what will happen to them. Let me now try to do something similar in delivering this book's key ideas. The setting is of our world being flooded with new information at an astonishing rate, one that is so rapid that many people describe *necessary* learning as trying to drink out of a fire hose. Since we cannot begin to deal with all the new information and knowledge that is available, how can we make better use of relevant portions?

In this regard, I have a burning desire: I want you to fulfill more of your God-given potential while applying the spiritual gifts and abilities that He has given you. I hope you will feel more of His heart for doing so as you read this book.

Here is a preview. We start in Part One: Breakthrough Learning Fundamentals by considering six fundamental elements of breakthrough learning, fundamentals that are too often ignored. Lesson One: Grasp the Discipline's Approach looks at the methods used by a discipline (a proven way of organizing and applying information) to solve problems and apply remedies. Some people describe disciplines from an academic perspective, closely matching them to various fields of study. Thus, chemists do different things to obtain truth than do art historians. In the rush to gain more information, learners in many disciplines may not have given sufficient attention to first identifying and mastering such approaches. Without such mastery, necessities of and limitations to the disciplines may not be properly understood. When there are misunderstandings, some mistakes will be made.

Lesson Two: Access Relevant Information looks at beginning to apply a discipline's approach. In some cases, doing so is merely a matter of sifting through the available information to selectively apply the right portions of the approach. All too often, however, relevant information needs to be developed before the approach can be applied. Breakthrough learning is especially likely to occur whenever valuable new information is developed, studied, and applied. Yet most people have learned little and appreciate still less about noticing when such information development is necessary and how to accomplish it.

In Lesson Three: Apply Chunks of Information and Knowledge, we consider how to overcome some limitations of our brains and nervous systems. The point is simple: If we try to do too many things at once, we will make mistakes, often grow frustrated, and may eventually quit trying. However, the same task, when broken down into simpler chunks, can be easily accomplished ... leading to accomplishing more and also feeling encouraged to do even more.

We have all seen "facts" that have been long accepted as true shown to be totally wrong by experiments, new information, and better analysis. Because of such rapid improvement in knowledge, we need to spend more time staying current, and Lesson Four looks into highly effective ways of doing so.

Lesson Five explains how to better apply knowledge to information. Many educational researchers have reported that only a tiny percentage of college graduates can correctly apply the disciplines they studied to address an everyday problem. In many cases, the limitation exists because these students had too little experience solving practical problems while learning the discipline. Without sufficient experience, they are then likely to make mistakes in solving everyday problems due to forgetting aspects of what's required, picking wrong methods, and focusing on the wrong information — mistakes that lead them to draw wrong conclusions. Such errors represent the best case. Most college graduates will, instead, just scratch their heads while failing to think of anything useful to do first, having forgotten most of what had been learned. However, when sufficient application experience has occurred during initial learning, any later loss of such skill can be quickly remedied.

Lesson Six concludes this first part by considering the enormous learning advantages of teaching others to effectively apply a discipline. While doing so, great strides are usually made by the instructor in understanding how each aspect of the discipline relates to each other one. By developing simpler and more effective ways to explain and demonstrate what is required, the people teaching can deepen and widen their understanding of what works and doesn't in applying the discipline.

Each of the book's three parts (Breakthrough Learning Fundamentals, Teach Yourself, and Teach Others) is preceded by a brief introduction containing an overview of the lessons to follow. I encourage you to read and think about these introductions before beginning the lessons to obtain a better foundation and framework for applying what you are learning.

Since introductions of the parts are available, let me much more briefly describe parts two and three than I did for Part One. However, if you don't feel you need to know this information now, skip ahead to read the introduction to Part One.

There is perhaps no more valuable skill for gaining personal benefits and serving others than becoming adept at learning new disciplines on one's own. In Part Two: Teach Yourself, we focus on the most important aspects of this form of learning. The material is divided into nine lessons that describe how to be highly effective in self-directed learning. Lesson Seven leads learners to find and study descriptions of the discipline's approach. After that, Lesson Eight explains how to identify the required skills for using this approach. Lesson Nine explores goal setting for applying the discipline. In Lesson Ten, we look at developing skills in chunks small enough to be easily absorbed, remembered, and applied. After that, learners can use Lesson Eleven to become adept in an effective process through focusing on the right-sized chunks for taking the necessary steps. As

Introduction

learners apply the discipline, Lesson Twelve describes how to measure performance while doing so and how to have someone check the learner's application of a discipline. Lesson Thirteen then directs the learner to improve the process that has just been used. In Lesson Fourteen, we consider the best ongoing ways to become aware of relevant new information and knowledge. Finally, Lesson Fifteen describes how to teach others and after that to stay up-to-date in the discipline and the best ways to teach it.

In Part Three: Teach Others, we look at instructing others so they quickly become highly effective breakthrough learners. Lesson Sixteen explains how to assist learners to develop their goals. Lesson Seventeen focuses on explaining a discipline's approach and how to apply it. Next, in Lesson Eighteen, you will discover effective ways to test learners for identifying what necessary skills, if any, they lack. Subsequently, Lesson Nineteen discusses how to demonstrate multiple ways of learning any needed skills. Lesson Twenty explains how to direct learners to practice applying the new skills so that their enhanced capabilities become permanent. In Lesson Twenty-One, we evaluate how to adjust the method for developing skills so that it will be more effective for future learners. Lesson Twenty-Two shows how to demonstrate application of the discipline to the learner's goals. In Lesson Twenty-Three, we describe how to observe and correct the learner's applications of the discipline to his or her goals. From there, Lesson Twenty-Four provides valuable insights into measuring, identifying, and addressing any underlying causes of errors and slowness. In Lesson Twenty-Five, we explain how to direct a learner to self-improve the process that she or he has been applying. Lesson Twenty-Six demonstrates the ways learners should be taught to update their awareness of important new information and knowledge. Finally, in Lesson Twenty-Seven, you are directed to repeat and improve upon the steps you have just applied while teaching still other learners.

In the book's Afterword, I spell out some important implications of what you have been learning. I also encourage you to read my personal testimony of how I came to follow Jesus as my Lord and Savior and how that relationship has improved my life, as well as a brief summary of The 400 Year Project, both of which are found in the appendixes.

As you can well imagine, the topics of these 27 lessons could easily become so abstract that you, my precious reader, might be puzzled by what to do. I have done my best to avoid that problem by providing examples that demonstrate in practical ways how you can become a breakthrough learner and assist others to do the same. To make the learning easier, you will also find stories that teach the lessons at a deeper level. Pay close attention to those stories. Mull them over in quiet moments. They will guide you in unexpected, powerful ways. Also, stay in prayer asking for the guidance of the Holy Spirit.

If after reading *Breakthrough Learning* you have questions, comments, or suggestions, I would be delighted to hear from you. My e-mail address is donmitchell@fastforward400.com/.

Let's turn now to the introduction of Part One.

Part One:

Breakthrough Learning Fundamentals

*Therefore, leaving the discussion of
the elementary principles of Christ,
let us go on to perfection, not laying again
the foundation of repentance from
dead works and of faith toward God,
of the doctrine of baptisms, of laying on of hands,
of resurrection of the dead, and of eternal judgment.
And this we will do if God permits.*

— Hebrews 6:1-3 (NKJV)

God created us to learn. While we are born with some hard-wired abilities, such as being able to breathe, suck, swallow, and open the eyes, most of the rest of the new infant's brain is little developed. Based on what experiences the baby later has, what information is received, and how the experiences and information are interpreted, learning begins. And our learning never ends. New neural connections are still being formed at the moment of our deaths.

While such learning is often seemingly accidental and undirected, keep in mind that God has a unique purpose for each life. Fulfilling that purpose requires that someone develop faith in God, something we are not born with, and then learn to apply that faith in fruitful ways. While many churches do a fine job of helping people come to faith and then assisting them to develop ways of drawing closer to God and of engaging in their callings from Him, I have yet to find a church (or any school, for that matter) that systematically demonstrates and teaches how to be the most effective possible doer of God's will.

While it's certainly tempting for me to write about all of the helpful ways of fruitfully applying Godly learning that are already in use, those topics are not within the scope of what this book addresses. However, I assume that you have already received some solid indications of what God is calling you to do for expanding and improving His Kingdom. If you have yet to receive a sense of that calling, I urge you to seek spiritual counsel so that you can begin to obtain this understanding. A pastor at your church will probably be happy to direct you to resources and to help you think through how God has formed you and what He has been doing to develop you through your relationship with Him.

If your experience with God has been like mine, you've been aware of His calling on your life for some time. As a result, you've been busily doing God's work. While faithfully serving, you have probably noticed that the focus of His calling for you has shifted (and possibly expanded) after following His directions. As the parables of the Minas (Luke 19:11-27, NKJV — a partial quotation can be found in Lesson Twenty-Seven) and of the Talents (Matthew 25:14-30, NKJV) indicate, God rewards those who make good use of time, resources, and skills. In response, He provides added opportunities and resources to accomplish more.

During your faith journey, God has probably asked you to do some pretty unbelievable things, things that stretched your faith by requiring you to rely more on Him. If you have not yet had such experiences, it's highly likely you eventually will. Relying more on Him and thereby gaining more faith are wonderful parts of being a believer, and they are also the best ways to accomplish more for Him.

You might wonder why I'm making such a point about relying on God in a book about becoming a more capable learner. My reason is a simple, but important, one: I want you to use *Breakthrough Learning* not to become more independent of God, but, rather, to become *more* dependent on Him to gain the results that He seeks from your efforts.

How might greater dependence on Him allow you to gain more benefits through applying *Breakthrough Learning*? One possibility is that by becoming a better learner Jesus will then be able to use you to produce more fruitful results. For instance, becoming a better learner can cause you to stand more in awe and appreciation of the One who provides the sources of the learning, as well as the supernatural assistance that can enable applying that learning to accomplish vastly more than anyone could ask, think, or imagine. After having such an experience, you'll become a more powerful witness to the fact that He is alive and with us. In addition, you'll be prepared to take on still more for Him, further enhancing your potential fruitfulness.

Deep down, everyone knows many of her or his individual limitations. Seeing others who are more talented in certain ways can deepen our reluctance to try new things that seem out of our own reach. For instance, because of my poor singing voice, I don't think about trying out for the church choir. Unfortunately, such a reaction can cause a harmful complacency. For example, God could have intended that my poor singing voice would encourage me to take lessons, lessons that will make me more fruitful in ways that I don't perceive but He intends. For instance, He may want me to witness to my singing teacher. When complacency reigns, we are often satisfied to merely observe those who can do remarkable things, enjoying their skill and vicariously experiencing their success while silently folding our arms in comfort. Such is the basis of fandom, something that's quite popular now.

While it can be usefully humbling for someone to know that he or she is limited and to appreciate what someone else can do better, searching for the remarkable should be first directed towards God, rather than towards paying attention to differently talented humans. In this part of *Breakthrough Learning*, I pray that you will be moved to see learning as coming from God for the purposes of drawing you closer to Him and of serving Him more effectively in expanding and improving His Kingdom.

If you find yourself focusing otherwise in the future, I strongly encourage you to reread this introduction to Part One.

As the Introduction more thoroughly explains and discusses, this part of *Breakthrough Learning* focuses on identifying and describing the most important elements of any kind of learning. Master these six lessons, and you'll avoid most of the mistakes that can make it difficult and frustrating to learn and apply what is studied. Let's turn now to Lesson One: Grasp the Discipline's Approach.

Lesson One:

Grasp the Discipline's Approach

Do you not know that those who run in a race all run,
but one receives the prize?
Run in such a way that you may obtain it.
And everyone who competes for the prize
is temperate in all things.
Now they do it to obtain a perishable crown,
but we for an imperishable crown.
Therefore I run thus: not with uncertainty.
Thus I fight: not as one who beats the air.
But I discipline my body and bring it into subjection,
lest, when I have preached to others,
I myself should become disqualified.

— 1 Corinthians 9:24-27 (NKJV)

Until writing this lesson, I had never considered the Apostle Paul's words in 1 Corinthians 9:24-27 (NKJV) as advice that is applicable for learning and teaching. However, such applications leapt into my mind as I reread these verses while writing this lesson. Let me explain what I mean in the context of someone who is preparing to run a marathon (a race covering a total distance of 26 miles and 385 yards, equal to 42.195 kilometers).

Most people would prepare for a marathon by training, rather than by just going out one day and running a race of that distance for the first time. Certainly, faster results should follow from first building endurance and strength rather than by starting without developing much of either one. If winning a prize was the goal, quite a bit of training might be necessary.

However, imagine what would happen if such a runner decided to train by only running backwards. While doing so would surely build a lot of endurance and strength due to the difficulty and effort involved, some muscles would be strengthened in the wrong ways for when running forward would be faster. Training for a marathon by running backwards can create similar effects to learners studying a discipline without having first understood the approach that would work best for applying it.

My first experience in this regard came as quite a shock: receiving a grade of "D" for my first college geology report. We had visited some rock outcroppings and had been told to identify the rocks and describe the conditions that had probably created what we observed. By using various tests (such as appearance, color, hardness, and reactions to acid), it was quite easy to accomplish the identifications. The part about the prior conditions was a little harder, but the answer was soon fairly clear.

I was feeling pretty pleased with myself about my work on the assignment until receiving that D. At my college, hardly anyone ever received such a low grade. My sole clue as to what I had done wrong was a handwritten note saying that I had used deductive logic (which means beginning with premises assumed to be true and then determining what else would have to be true) rather than inductive logic (deriving conclusions after exhaustively analyzing data) to develop my answers.

If that note on my lab report makes limited sense to you now, at the time it didn't make any more sense to me. After speaking with the grader, I came to appreciate that my task in applying geology was to maximize the application of *all* the evidence to draw my conclusions, rather than to string deductive logic together by using the minimum of empirical evidence. While the latter approach is often applauded as being "elegant" and desirable in a mathematical proof based on axioms, in geology doing so was a no-no. Who knew? I certainly didn't.

From this example, you can easily see that every learner needs to know how truth is sought and ascertained in a given discipline. Otherwise, learning will be less fruitful and easily avoidable mistakes will be made. If you are wondering why I am making a big point about doing so, think about any experiences you've had with someone patiently describing to you what needed to be done to solve a problem ... but having what was said make little sense to you. Such impenetrable explanations are often based on deep, unstated understandings of how truth is sought and proven. The person explaining the points has often absorbed many of such understandings indirectly through considering the works of many others in the field. As another potential complication in gaining understanding, explanations are often couched in technical terms whose meanings are different in the context of that field than in a nontechnical, everyday conversation. Further, someone who frequently works in the field may expect that everyone else understands the discipline's assumptions, while the struggling learner may recognize little, if anything, about the reasons for what is seen or heard.

I was reminded of this last difficulty about expectations just yesterday while helping a student prepare for a college entrance examination. She became completely confused by the explanation for the correct answer in the "official" guide, which had no doubt been written by quite capable experts. In this particular case, the explanation assumed that the student already understood by inspection of the problem that the two sides of the equation differed only in that one side was the result of dividing the other side by the factor found in the denominator of the fraction on that side of the equation. Although she had studied math for many years and was good at solving problems, as best she could remember this was the first time she had been exposed to this kind of a problem or explanation. If written in

Lesson One: Grasp the Discipline's Approach

Sanskrit, the explanation would have been just about as helpful to this student who knew no Sanskrit.

So *what should you do?* If you are fortunate enough to find someone knowledgeable in the discipline who is well aware of and able to clearly articulate the approaches and assumptions involved, then your pathway is clear. Just ask. Realize that in some cases you may have to pay for such help, but the benefits will usually be well worth the cost. You will gain much effectiveness by having taken the time to do so. Most other would-be learners will decide to skip this essential step, simply because no one has explained to them how valuable this step can be.

However, you are more than likely not to find such a person ... at best locating someone who can only spell out part of what you need to learn. When that's the case, this first lesson can help by outlining some questions you should ask of those with partial knowledge about what you need to learn.

First, *how are deductive and inductive forms of reasoning used to determine truth in this discipline?* While many experts will quickly assert that only one or the other form of reasoning is used, be skeptical of such answers and press forward for more details. Most disciplines employ both kinds of reasoning to some degree for accomplishing quite different purposes. For instance, while many sciences build a knowledge base from observing appropriate evidence in detail and then generalizing from it, the same sciences often apply mathematics and other methods that rely on deductive reasoning for part of the analysis. While applications of law, as a different example, are often deduced from prior cases and long-established legal principles, in individual cases judges have thrown out precedent that didn't square with well-done and quite complete empirical studies of what is happening in similar current situations. The school-desegregation decision in *Brown v. Board of Education of Topeka*, 347 U.S. 483 (1954) in the United States is such an example. Precedent had previously ruled that schools could be racially segregated if they were equal in providing for students. The plaintiffs used empirical evidence in *Brown* to show that such separate schools could never be equal. The Supreme Court justices were persuaded by this evidence and overturned the precedent.

Without knowing how the two kinds of reasoning blend together, you'll be quick to make mistakes. I often see such errors being made by people who love the Bible. Their knowledge may be so complete that they can find a single passage to "prove" almost anything. While doing so, such individuals can fall into the trap of extrapolating from a single verse to draw a major conclusion. Most Bible scholars agree that you should, instead, apply all verses that relate to the subject, either directly or indirectly, and also consider the context for each verse. Quite different conclusions will often follow from doing so.

Second, *what mistakes are most likely to occur when applying deductive and/or inductive reasoning in this discipline?* Most people who are familiar with a discipline can describe some occasions when errors have been made that were later corrected. After some discussion with such a person, the two of you should be able to pin down the major sources of such mistakes. In many disciplines, including unstated assumptions that represent contemporary values often lead to such errors. Thus, most people who write about political science tacitly assume that just some people should have certain rights when penning seemingly universal statements, while never actually mentioning that those grand statements do not apply to everyone in all ways. The U.S. Constitution was written, for instance, on the assumption that slaves were merely property, rather than human beings, while stating all kinds of valuable rights for citizens. In those times, despite women being identified as human, they then had limited rights based on unstated assumptions reflecting then commonly held beliefs.

Third, *how can mistakes be avoided when applying deductive and inductive reasoning in this discipline?* While many disciplines require review by experts before conclusions are accepted, such reviews can be tainted by insufficient knowledge, inadequate attention, carelessness, cultural assumptions, and self-interest. For these reasons, improving the review process can be very valuable. Some scientific disciplines, for instance, require that any new "truth" be disclosed in sufficient detail that someone else can repeat what was done and obtain the same results. For instance, in the aftermath of extravagant reports about accomplishing so-called cold fusion that gripped the world's attention for a bit, this kind of review process prevented a serious misunderstanding from occurring when others could not duplicate the reported results.

Fourth, *what is the intersection of this discipline with other disciplines?* As a law student, I took a course in how the law treats mental illness for which a law professor and a physician served as instructors. Before taking the class, I expected that they would have melded the two fields together. Instead, their two approaches seemed to be headed off on totally different trajectories into infinity, ones that would never intersect unless redirected. However, the good news is that many disciplines are now expanding to develop approaches that combine with at least one other discipline. A good example can be found at Harvard University where different faculties have been encouraged to collaborate for advancing understanding of the brain. While the medical school is obviously involved, so are the schools of public health and education. When such academic connections are developed, they can operate in ways similar to how the neural connections in a single brain combine different experiences, memories, and perspectives to develop useful unified perceptions, decisions, and actions.

Fifth, *what is the discipline ignoring?* While those in all disciplines feel that they are close to or are actually putting a literal finger on the truth, such knowledge is usually accurate only from a narrow perspective, a less valuable viewpoint than any one that encompasses more dimensions over time. For instance, how much can you understand about feeling love by only reading a description of how the body's chemistry changes while just being near to someone else? As a different example, I particularly remember being surprised by how little attention my law school courses paid to justice from either God's or society's perspective. I had arrived in law school with the mistaken idea that law was primarily a way of seeking and providing justice. Instead, classes mostly focused on correctly applying what a majority of legislators had voted for, laws that typically reflected awkward compromises made by political factions that had been considerably influenced by special interests, rather than by looking into how to provide justice.

Sixth, *what questions cannot be answered by this discipline?* You may find differences of opinion on this subject. Some advocates may argue that the discipline can answer almost anything. Others from the same discipline may argue, instead, that very few things can be answered. Some critics of the discipline may suggest that even less can be known. The truth will often lie somewhere between the extremes. The value of this question can be found in becoming appropriately cautious about stretching a discipline beyond where it fits well.

Seventh, *where is the discipline starving for a lack of better information?* We are fortunate to live in an age when information can be more easily and completely developed than ever before. While many people assume that the digital age has mainly affected communications and scientific disciplines, almost every discipline has been improved, in part, by being able to quantify things that were previously impractical to characterize in such a way. For instance, the simple pie charts that often illustrate today's history texts were often missing a few decades ago because of the impractical amount of work required then to compile the data. Being aware of where there are data insufficiencies will also help you to take a more careful approach to the "knowledge" that has been distilled in these areas. Much like the "canals" that astronomers first thought they saw on Mars while peering through simple telescopes, some of such "knowledge" may also prove to be an illusion.

Eighth, *what skills must be used and how should they be correctly applied to the discipline?* While many people take for granted that anyone engaged in a discipline has all the proper skills, such may not be the case. I more frequently see this difficulty when two disciplines rely on one another. I ran into an example while helping one of my students prepare a textbook about properly using math to identify where oil and gas might be found beneath the Earth's surface. Prior to the textbook's creation, many petroleum geologists used math to misapply data in ways that created errors in choosing where to drill, leading to many unnecessary and expensive "dry" holes.

Ninth, *where can appropriate information and skills be efficiently accessed by those who lacking in either or both?* If all of us had to become experts in everything, I fear that very little useful advancement of knowledge and effectiveness would occur. In many cases, we just have a one-time need. In at least such instances, it will be more helpful to properly apply the discipline by simply getting appropriate help. A lot more breakthroughs are going to occur when that approach is taken. Most disciplinary experts are easily able to point out useful sources of help and information. In fact, I'm sure I've done so thousands of times to answer questions about the disciplines that I happen to understand.

Tenth, *what questions have I not asked that would greatly help me to correctly understand and apply this discipline?* It's pure arrogance to think that any set of questions (especially mine here) will reveal all of what should be understood and applied concerning a discipline. Be sure to open the conversation at some point to learn whatever someone more knowledgeable feels you should be sure to know ... but you didn't know enough to ask questions about.

While no set of questions is going to uncover every possible bit of information and knowledge that you need for best applying a discipline, I'm sure that answering this set of questions will cause you to more frequently avoid the kind of error that I made on that long-ago geology report. However, do proceed cautiously. It never hurts to recheck your understanding of how to engage in a discipline before either taking any major steps to apply it or incurring significant expense.

Breakthrough Learning

Your Assignments

1. What disciplines should you learn to better apply your calling from God?

2. How are deductive and inductive forms of reasoning used to determine truth in each of these disciplines?

3. What mistakes are most likely to occur when applying deductive and inductive reasoning in these disciplines?

4. How can mistakes be avoided in applying deductive and inductive reasoning in these disciplines?

5. What are the useful intersections of these disciplines with other disciplines?

6. What is each discipline ignoring?

7. What questions cannot be answered by these disciplines?

8. Where are the disciplines starving for lack of better information?

9. What skills must be used and how should they be correctly applied to each of the disciplines?

10. Where can appropriate information and skills be efficiently accessed by those who are lacking in either or both for applying the disciplines?

11. What other information do you lack to correctly understand and apply these disciplines?

12. Who can help you correctly answer these questions?

Lesson Two:

Access Relevant Information

For through Him we both have access by one Spirit to the Father.

— Ephesians 2:18 (NKJV)

In addition to the increasing availability of information, please keep in mind that much of it could be used improperly. For instance, online sites often rank information based on how many people report that it has been "useful" to them. Information in such cases is being measured in the eye of the beholders, regardless of its objective accuracy or relevance to a specific other individual, such as you. These kinds of results can be misleading. For instance, if someone says something nice about one of my books, even if what is said isn't very helpful to anyone else, I will often feel that the comment has been "useful" from my perspective and so indicate. Someone may later choose to purchase a book that has been blessed with many such characterizations of positive online comments about the book that have been mostly made by authors, and their publishers, publicists, families, and friends. After receiving the book, the purchaser could potentially find it, in fact, to be irrelevant or useless for almost anyone.

Ephesians 2:18 (NKJV) refers to Jesus as the source of our ability to access our Heavenly Father through the Holy Spirit who resides in all believers. Such access is extremely important. First, God already knows everything that is true. Through access to Him, we can gain truth that is otherwise inaccessible. Second, because He loves

Lesson Two: Access Relevant Information

us, He will supply truth in just the ways that will be most helpful for our spiritual development, as well as for advancing His Kingdom. Consequently, I most highly recommend gaining access to relevant information through praying for God's guidance and then paying close attention to whatever directions are received. While He is perfect, we unfortunately aren't. So be sure to pray for His reaction to any conclusions you draw from such directions to ensure that you are actually going to do what He wants.

In the course of learning how a discipline should be applied, you will no doubt meet some people who are extremely knowledgeable about the work that has been and is now being done. As you begin to access information for applying whatever Godly directions you have received, check back with such individuals for help in finding the best related work that has been done in the field. As an example, I was fortunate to have an outstanding history tutor as a junior in college. One of my assignments then was to write a long research paper. While looking for a possible topic, I mentioned that I enjoyed doing new research more than evaluating research and analysis that others had done. The tutor then asked me what historical subjects I liked to study. I told him of my longstanding interest in railroads. I mentioned that my dad worked for one and that my main scholarship was being paid for by his employer. My tutor's eyes brightened, he snapped his fingers, and said, "We've just finished a major project reading French newspapers. We noticed that there were many reports of attacks on railroads in France during the two revolutions in 1848. Would you be interested in reading those reports and turning what you find into a research paper?" I jumped at the chance. Revolutions were then the only subject that I liked to study better than railroads. I was fascinated by how rapidly human attitudes and behaviors shifted during such times and wanted to learn more. I had just been directed to a dream assignment! Notice that I was very unlikely to have found this topic, a topic which kept me happily occupied for the next 18 months, without having had my experienced tutor's knowledge and timely help.

In most disciplines, online literature searches can usually be conducted by focusing on reputable outlets for new information and knowledge. While doing so, you can check to see what is and isn't known. While searches that employ key words can be helpful, I also encourage reading summaries of all the newer articles in the best outlets, some of which could have important relevance concerning perspectives to apply. In addition, you should look for any new research methods that can be applied to your topic. For the most part in such searches, stay focused on sources of information that have been validated in some way that's appropriate to the discipline. Otherwise, you'll be reading about "miracle" solutions whose results some public relations person exaggerated to gain attention. Many such "puff" pieces can be found even in some of the otherwise well-respected popular publications.

However, in some instances you will notice that a new form of analysis can be brought to bear on an old problem, one where many data are already available. Typically, such opportunities can be found in places where incomplete or only elementary analysis has been previously done, providing freedom to apply more powerful methods.

In such analyses, be cautious; many sources of so-called official information are not worth the paper they are printed on. Because of the great demand for information in many disciplines, governments and nonprofit institutes feel compelled to supply certain data. Due to the difficulty of properly doing so, pressure to come up with a pleasing answer, or lack of time and budget to do the job adequately, some of such provided "facts" are simply the result of applying incorrect assumptions to other sets of data. Such results may, in fact, bear little resemblance to reality.

As an example, consider the unemployment rate in the United States. This closely watched percentage is reported monthly. While many people assume that this figure is generated by counting all the people who used to have jobs but don't now, and then dividing the number of unemployed by the sum of how many people are unemployed and how many people have full-time jobs, such an assumption is far from the truth. Instead, many unemployed people are removed from the total after they stop looking for work because of becoming discouraged by a shortage of opportunities. For instance, many people in their sixties cannot find a new job due to their age and health. However, surveys report that many such people would like to work for at least a few more years. Despite this, such individuals who desire to work would not appear in the unemployed number after four weeks of being inactive in taking a job-seeking action. Yet if someone contacted one of these people with a good job offer, she or he would probably take it. Isn't that person really unemployed now? The employment total used in the denominator also differs from what you might think should be included. For instance, if you work at least 15 hours a week, you are considered to be employed ... even if you work for a family business and receive no pay. In addition, people with two jobs are usually counted as though two people were being employed, rather than one. I could go on to point other data oddities in calculating the unemployment rate, but I'm sure you get the idea: This rate is based on an arbitrary way to measure that understates the reality of involuntary joblessness.

While there may be some kind of information available that can be applied to your investigation, realize that it may not be relevant for what you want to do. If you run into that difficulty, don't be discouraged! In many cases, those who "massage" information for a given purpose may well have more fundamental data that you can access and use to answer your question. Ask the data managers for such raw detail. For instance, American economists often construct their own versions of the unemployment rate based, in part, on government data. I've seen times when such alternative calculations indicated an unemployment percentage more than four times the government-reported rate. As you can well appreciate, no government wants to give the impression that it is causing harm to people in the nation, and those in charge of preparing the reports have the power to change the measurement to create a more positive impression.

However, you are likely in at least some cases to find that there are not enough adequate data available. As an example, I first found studying ways to eliminate poverty to be quite challenging because there were few data that could be accessed. Existing data were also mostly at such aggregate levels and insufficiently complete to provide full understanding. When I tried to use cross-national data to draw conclusions by applying statistical methods, no useful insights were produced.

Rather than just feel frustrated, I thought about alternatives and realized that experiments could usefully develop insights. If experiments began to suggest ways that poverty could be eliminated, those answers, in turn, could inform developing new data to more helpfully record the circumstances and activities of poor people. While I didn't have any idea of how to conduct such experiments at the time, God later provided me with many graduate students whose experiments I was privileged to supervise. After many years, I began to see what kinds of data would be most valuable for measuring how well poor people were being assisted.

Hopefully, your learning task won't require as much groundwork before useful data are developed. To ensure progress in the near term, always pick your data-development goals with an eye to the related costs and difficulties. I have also found it helpful to share with others the methods for data development that I intend to use. In many cases, vastly more efficient ways of accomplishing the same result have been suggested, enabling data development to be accomplished faster, more completely, and at much less expense.

For the moment, bear with me while I briefly explain something that you probably know: the value of working with samples. To answer many questions, you don't have to measure everything. You just have to carefully measure a randomly selected sample of sufficient size. If you've never done so, these sentences may mean little to you. Let me be more specific. Having developed data about many forms of human behavior, I've been struck by how often a sample of between 100 and 1,500 has been sufficient to answer quite important

Lesson Two: Access Relevant Information

and challenging questions. While those numbers mean that there are still quite a few people or things to measure in the sample, doing so is certainly a lot easier than counting everything that's going on. In other words, samples allow us to scope down the amount of work that is required to an amount that is practical in all but those cases where measurement of each individual, thing, or circumstance in the sample is extremely expensive.

Since the cost of measuring can still be a limitation on learning more, let me address how to further reduce such costs in other ways. Keep in mind while making any cost reductions that the choice of measurement precision is important for two reasons. First, without sufficient precision, the results can be misleading. Second, adding precision exponentially increases the costs. So deciding how to measure should be based, in part, on a careful analysis of balancing sufficient precision with the costs of obtaining it. My experience with data development has been that many people stop too soon while considering how much precision they need. Such premature conclusions are often connected to believing that only one way of measuring can do the job, a method that's often the most obvious one. However, much in the way that geometry allows us to measure things that we cannot easily reach (such as determining the height of a tall tree by measuring the distance on the ground from the tree to the point where the top of the tree can be seen through a special angle, such as 30 or 45 degrees, and then applying the Pythagorean Theorem), you can often benefit by taking an indirect approach to data development.

Here's an example. Assume that you want to estimate the market potential for a new product. In quite a large country, doing so directly might mean constructing prototypes, providing them to a large random sample of potential customers and users, carefully observing what was done with the prototypes, and asking detailed questions about each person's reaction to the prototype. While doing so would give you quite a precise answer within the range of whatever the sample size permitted, this approach could also involve more work than is necessary. For instance, if there were, in fact, very little or extremely large market potential, obtaining either answer would have been sufficient to decide either to cancel the product's development or to continue developing it. How might indirect evidence be used to obtain such answers in such a case? One possibility is by looking to see if there's an existing offering of another type that presents somewhat comparable kinds of benefits, costs, and difficulties for customers and end users. If you can find such an offering, for drawing an accurate conclusion about your development project you might only need to know the approximate annual volumes purchased from the time of the earlier offering's introduction. If you could find several of such items, you could then combine the perspectives gained from each to add more precision to your gross estimate, while still keeping the costs of developing information quite low.

If you run into a data-development problem that you find to be difficult, feel free to contact me at donmitchell@fastforward400.com/. I may not know the answer, but perhaps I can at least point you further down the path towards a good one.

Your Assignments

1. What information is available to help you learn what you seek?

2. What are the limitations of such information?

3. What information would be most helpful?

4. Will it be necessary to develop any new information?

5. If new information is required, how precise do you need it to be?

6. What are the most time- and cost-efficient ways to obtain exactly the new information you need with the minimum precision required for sufficient accuracy?

Lesson Three:

Apply Chunks of Information and Knowledge

> *But the manifestation of the Spirit is given*
> *to each one for the profit* of all:
> *for to one is given the word of wisdom through the Spirit,*
> *to another the word of knowledge through the same Spirit,*
> *to another faith by the same Spirit,*
> *to another gifts of healings by the same Spirit,*
> *to another the working of miracles, to another prophecy,*
> *to another discerning of spirits,*
> *to another* different *kinds of tongues,*
> *to another the interpretation of tongues.*
> *But one and the same Spirit works all these things,*
> *distributing to each one individually as He wills.*
>
> — 1 Corinthians 12:7-11 (NKJV)

In 1 Corinthians 12:7-11 (NKJV), the Apostle Paul described how the Holy Spirit provides different spiritual gifts to believers. In doing so, Paul asserted that behind such provision is a plan for each believer to apply spiritual gifts in ways that will profit all. To appreciate the wisdom of such an approach, imagine a situation where *each* believer had been abundantly provided with *all* the spiritual gifts. How would a church decide who would deliver the messages, who

Lesson Three: Apply Chunks of Information and Knowledge

would make decisions about matters of greatest consequence, who would apply knowledge to solve problems, who would heal, who would work miracles, and so forth? If some of such applications of spiritual gifts were considered to be more attractive by many believers, a large number of people might vie to take on these roles. Whatever else occurred, I can easily imagine a congregation that would soon be divided into factions concerning ideas of what to do next or ways of making assignments to use spiritual gifts.

God's plan for us also shows other ways that being more focused is valuable. For instance, we are reminded that if we try to serve two masters, we will love one and hate the other (Matthew 6:24, NKJV). In the story of Mary and Martha in Luke 10:38-42 (NKJV), we also find encouragement to place our focus on Jesus, rather than only on doing things for Jesus.

In recent years, much has been learned (but just a tiny fraction of what it would be desirable to know) about how the brain functions. One of the most significant observations for breakthrough learning is that more can be accomplished by most people if they pay attention to just one thing at a time. As I considered that finding, I was surprised to realize that what I had often thought of as doing *multitasking* in my own work is not that at all. Instead, I merely rotate total focus from one thing to another when I need a break from whatever I am doing at the moment. For instance, I might be drafting this book, but stop for two minutes to look out the window at a bird after hearing it chirp. After tiring of watching the bird, but not yet being ready to write more, I might then check my e-mails.

True multitasking looks like this instead: While typing words to draft this book, I might be simultaneously speaking to someone on the telephone, watching out the window for a delivery van to arrive, and mentally planning a reunion celebration with high school classmates. I don't know about you, but I would make a mess out of each thing while simultaneously trying to do so many tasks. A more capable person would do better than I would, but the results would still be less than if a singular focus had been applied.

We also have another limitation that's worthwhile considering. Short-term memory capacity is small. This limitation is one reason why telephone numbers don't have more digits. In the days before many people carried a cellphone that kept track of telephone numbers, most people relied on their memories to recall such numbers while away from home. If telephone numbers had too many digits, the total set of numbers would usually just seem to slip away from the mind. Here's why: Each time another number is added to your overloaded short-term memory, a number is dropped. You can test this out by writing down a 15-digit number. Look at it for 10 seconds, and then try to remember it 2 hours later. Unless the number is expressed in some simple pattern such as sequentially, you probably won't be able to do so. Do the same with a random 5-digit number, and you'll probably succeed.

So what's the point? If we break down tasks into smaller pieces (what I like to call "chunks"), accomplishing the tasks becomes exponentially easier and faster. Here's an example. Imagine that I give you an instruction to perform a task that goes like this: Use the attached sheet to find the cost of goods sold, subtract the result from the selling price to obtain the gross margin, then divide the new result into the total cost of investment to find how many units must be sold to break even, and next determine what market share that number of units represents.

Chances are that your head is swimming just a bit.

Let me break the same task down into chunks. Here's the first chunk. I want you to find the gross margin as measured in dollars for a single unit of this product. To do so, multiply the gross margin percentage (20 percent as a decimal, 0.2) by the selling price ($1,340). The answer to the first chunk is $268.

We move on to the second chunk. The total cost of the investment is $130,000,000. Divide $130,000,000 by $268. The answer to the second chunk is that 485,075 units are needed to break even.

We are now ready for the third chunk. Divide 485,075 units by 3,600,000 market units to obtain the market share represented by

Lesson Three: Apply Chunks of Information and Knowledge

the break-even number of units. The answer to the third chunk is 13.5 percent.

Now, wasn't the chunk approach a lot easier to think about and more helpful for doing this task?

This example is based on an actual problem assigned in an MBA program. Because the instructions read more like the first version, a student made grievous errors that would have doomed his grade. After I broke the work down into these chunks that included an example, he then correctly completed four pages of calculations in about 7 minutes, far less time than when he did the work incorrectly based on the original instructions. He later reported that the average grade in his class on this assignment was near 70 percent.

More significantly, in applying the chunks the student gained confidence that he could do this work quite effectively. When I then suggested various other ways he could prepare for the next assignments, he readily agreed to do so. He had gone from feeling puzzled and awkward to being aware that he understood exactly what to do and could easily be counted on to do so in the future.

While some would correctly point out that the first set of instructions in this lesson didn't provide the relevant numbers to perform the calculations, please consider that the student's assignment sheet contained five pages of numbers, from which he was expected to find just the appropriate few numbers to do the task. Understandably, he had picked some of the wrong numbers. In other cases, he misapplied the correct numbers. I don't want to waste your time by having you crawl through 5 pages of such information, so I omitted that part of the example. After understanding this point, I am sure you are even more aware of the benefits of turning tasks into smaller chunks that are easier to understand and perform.

In the case of this MBA student, a one-time task was given by the professor for the purpose of developing a basic skill. Naturally, doing that one assignment is not enough to master the skill.

Let's look at how chunks can lead to mastery. Notice that by first doing the task in chunks, it will be relatively easy for the student to then make his own notes about what is required to do each of the chunks. He can then rapidly build skill by repeating the chunks using slightly different numbers. After some number of repetitions of such drills with various other sets of numbers, the student would be in a good position to recall in the future how to accomplish the entire task. His memory would be built around performing those chunks, much in the way that a homebuilder first thinks about digging a hole for the foundation before doing any other building work, such as by putting in the forms to contain concrete for constructing the home's foundation.

While repeating chunks in relevant variations to develop such skill, much more difficult chunks than are presented in this example can be mastered more easily when practice is confined to a single chunk before moving on to practice the next chunk. For instance, if someone is learning to read social-science essays to notice the logical steps in the argument, the sources of evidence, and the appropriateness of the examples used, such an individual should just practice noticing one of those three areas before moving on to practice noticing a different one.

While I may seem to be belaboring an obvious point, please realize that the value of focusing narrowly must not be very obvious. Why? Because when I review the most popular texts in use on standard subjects, I rarely see any attempts to chunk tasks into simple pieces. And I never see a sufficient number of practice assignments to enable any but the most able students to actually master what's needed. Instead, the emphasis seems to be on how many topics can be covered in less and less time. By increasing the number of topics, the potential for confusing the learner grows exponentially. That potential for problems is especially true in disciplines that build on prior learning when adding new topics. Confuse a learner at the early stages, and he or she will be lost for the duration.

Once lost in knowing what to do, a student's morale drops. The student starts to see herself or himself as a loser in this subject. Having helped many students go from having such despair to stardom in

Lesson Three: Apply Chunks of Information and Knowledge

their disciplines, I know that it takes about 10 times more effort to help such a confused learner than to teach the discipline in chunks from the beginning. So be good to yourself and others, and learn in small chunks. You will move faster and more accurately if you do. You'll also feel much more encouraged to learn the next thing.

<u>Your Assignments</u>

1. How can you concentrate on learning so it will occur with the fewest distractions?

2. What are the steps involved to acquire the new learning and to apply it in practice?

3. How can each step be broken down into simpler, easier-to-understand chunks?

4. How can you vary how each chunk is performed with different facts or applications so that you can repeat the chunk often enough to master the tasks involved in it?

5. When will you practice to maintain your mastery?

Lesson Four:

Update Information and Knowledge

"No one sews a piece of unshrunk cloth on an old garment;
or else the new piece pulls away from the old,
and the tear is made worse.
And no one puts new wine into old wineskins;
or else the new wine bursts the wineskins,
the wine is spilled, and the wineskins are ruined.
But new wine must be put into new wineskins."

— Mark 2:21-22 (NKJV)

In Mark 2:21-22 (NKJV), Jesus answered a question about why His disciples did not fast while those of John and the Pharisees did. He went on to predict that the disciples would fast after He was gone from them. He likened the time while He was with them to when friends celebrate the marriage of a new bridegroom. It was a time for rejoicing rather than fasting.

Similarly, we have all had the experience of gaining new information, knowledge, or experience that left us feeling on top of the world, such as when believers first begin to follow Jesus as their Lord and Savior. Such a feeling, while wonderful, can also lull us into a false sense of complacency. If that once-stimulating information and knowledge becomes obsolete due to changed condi-

Lesson Four: Update Information and Knowledge

tions, we become, in effect, the equivalent of an old garment or an old wineskin. We either need to have new information and knowledge pre-shrunk to fit us as old garments, or we need to be transformed by the new information and knowledge so that we can be like new wineskins.

You are probably wondering how to be sure that we stay current in information and knowledge. Of course, any such updating has to be done efficiently, or we will have little time to accomplish anything else.

The best updating methods vary widely from discipline to discipline. Begin by asking people who have long been involved in the discipline how often significant changes occur in either information or knowledge. In fairly stable disciplines such as those related to an earlier literary period, the answer may be that important changes seldom occur. In fast-developing scientific disciplines, such as those related to genetic engineering, such changes may occur very frequently.

Also ask experts to identity the most reliable sources of new information and knowledge. In addition, ask how best to work with such sources. In some cases, a useful publication may be scanned. In other cases, you might need to speak with someone who edits the publication, someone whose work requires staying up-to-date with much of the best new information and knowledge. Sometimes the cost of doing so is no more than buying breakfast or lunch. Some knowledgeable people are even happy to help all who make an occasional telephone call.

However, keep in mind that almost all disciplines ignore some of the most significant new sources of information and knowledge. Because that's true, you should also access unconventional sources ... especially those that are strongly rejected by the discipline's established authorities. For instance, near the end of a conversation with an expert you might gently ask about what "new" sources of information and knowledge have recently been rejected and the reasons for doing so. In assessing what you hear, keep in mind that disciplines generally become more sophisticated and refined over time.

As that development occurs, there's often a tendency to reject alternative approaches that are simpler, arise from a different perspective, or don't require much sophistication or refinement. However, such changes often become ones that sweep aside the more sophisticated and refined approaches due to their being easier and less costly to apply. Be especially curious about sources that might be developing in such directions.

I find it valuable to visit those who have created the greatest controversy and rejection to hear what they have to say about what the more traditional people are doing in the discipline. From such interactions, I often obtain a more objective sense of what's valuable and what's not among new information and knowledge than I do from those who operate in the ways that most people accept.

My great mentor, Peter Drucker, was one such valuable source. Peter was always very interested in gaining new perspectives and in challenging conventional wisdom. To do so, he sought to come at problems and situations from an objective, unbiased perspective that operated outside of any given discipline. He favored creating solutions by applying aspects of as many disciplines as possible ... and trying to find even more aspects of different disciplines to apply. Adding perspectives, in his view, was essential to learning more of what you need to know.

One way he gained an independent and unique perspective was by intensely investigating a new discipline each year. In choosing the discipline, he delighted in being eclectic. He also had no particular agenda in mind for gaining practical benefits. Yet, he told me that sometimes the best new insights came from the sources others might consider unlikely to provide any practical benefits. For example, he gained great understanding of management from Japanese print making, a discipline that few such experts would have thought to explore and apply.

Also check if new methods make it possible to gain information in cost-effective ways for the first time. In this regard, I often find it helpful to work with professors and professionals who offer services

Lesson Four: Update Information and Knowledge

involving new methods. From doing so, I gain access to their experiences, as well as to their technical knowledge about what can be done. While with them, I describe what I would like to learn and then delineate scenarios of how I perceive that these new methods might be applied in such a way. While I sometimes hit on a real possibility that's worth exploring, more often the reaction to my scenario is barely restrained amusement. Then, after that happens, I am gently let down with an explanation of why my imagined opportunity doesn't exist. But that's okay. I'd rather have my imagination get carried away with an impractical idea that I learn not to implement than miss a practical opportunity to gain valuable new information and knowledge.

If the discipline holds occasional conferences where researchers present their newest work, attending such meetings can be extremely valuable for staying up-to-date in rapidly developing disciplines. Many of the presentations will describe work that isn't yet published. In addition, speakers are often generous in explaining why they did or didn't choose to apply certain methods, information, and knowledge. Such speakers are often quite willing to talk informally about their personal wish lists for what they would like to explore if only some constraint or other were removed.

Simultaneously, such conferences provide many informal opportunities to have conversations with other attendees. In most cases, the conference coordinators will make available a list of attendees. When possible, I scan such lists in advance of attending. If time permits, I will invite several people who interest me to have breakfast, lunch, or dinner at a time that doesn't conflict with the conference program. Most people are flattered to be invited and arrive expecting to "sing for their supper" a bit by sharing what's on their minds. I try to have gained enough knowledge about what they or their organizations are doing so that I can ask relevant questions designed to illuminate possible new information and knowledge. In doing so, I avoid compromising their integrity and loyalty. I don't want to access their secrets. I just want to find out if there's something new that's worth tracking down. Most people are quite properly unwilling to tell any secrets, but they are often happy to suggest whether a search for information and knowledge is likely to be a useful activity.

I have also found it valuable to be a reviewer of new books in disciplines that interest me. Such reviews are usually about books I would have read anyway. Writing the review takes relatively little time and provides me with a convenient set of notes for refreshing my memory in the future about the book's contents. Each published review in a discipline will eventually attract the attention of several authors who would like to learn what I think of their books, and they will usually send free copies to make it easier. If I find an author I like, I encourage a relationship, which then provides me with more potential access to new information and knowledge.

As you can see, comfortable and easy ways to update information and knowledge will vary quite a bit from individual to individual and from discipline to discipline. I have provided examples of what has worked for me, but many of such activities might not appeal or make sense to you in terms of the disciplines on which you are focused. So please treat my described possibilities as being nothing more than a place to start your thinking about how to update information and knowledge. Be sure to let serendipity play a role, as well!

Your Assignments

1. In what aspects of the disciplines that interest you are new information and knowledge likely to be most valuable?

2. What are good sources of obtaining new information and knowledge concerning these aspects soon after they are developed?

3. How would it be most convenient and comfortable for you to connect with these sources?

Lesson Four: Update Information and Knowledge

4. Who could help you find even better sources and ways to gain new information and knowledge from them?

5. How can you best gain such assistance?

Lesson Five:

Apply the Discipline

And behold, a certain lawyer stood up and tested Him, saying, "Teacher, what shall I do to inherit eternal life?"

He said to him, "What is written in the law? What is your reading of it?"

So he answered and said, "'You shall love the L<small>ORD</small> your God with all your heart, with all your soul, with all your strength, and with all your mind,' and 'your neighbor as yourself.'"

And He said to him, "You have answered rightly; do this and you will live."

— Luke 10:25-28 (NKJV)

Luke 10:25-28 (NKJV) contains the conversation that led Jesus to tell the Parable of the Good Samaritan. Like the lawyer speaking to Jesus in these verses, learning about a discipline or a means of doing things can seem quite natural and appealing ... until we realize that we have to begin applying what we've been learning. Instead of feeling comfortable, we can quickly feel unprepared and disquieted. Af-

Lesson Five: Apply the Discipline

ter having this reaction, we often ask questions about how to avoid whatever seems threatening or unpleasant to us. In the case of the lawyer, he wanted to find out who his neighbor was. Possibly he was hoping that Jesus would answer that there were few people that the lawyer needed to love as much as he did himself. Wrong!

Many learners never comprehend what it means to competently apply a given discipline they have studied. In reality, many learners confuse competence in applying a given discipline with earning a good grade in a course covering some aspect of the discipline. Also wrong! Competently applying a given discipline requires solving an important problem or accomplishing something significant in a way that would not be possible without accurate knowledge and skill.

The issue of competence often arises during my graduate-school teaching. Students sometimes propose I teach a custom course that involves their reading about something and then describing how the reading's materials would have directed them to have done something different in some past situation or circumstance. While I think that such a focus is fine as far as it goes, I always tell them they will learn a great deal more by also applying the knowledge gained from the reading and evaluation of past experiences to a present task or challenge. Invariably, students agree and go on to do some very fine work. In many cases, they also learn important lessons about themselves. For instance, one student was very interested in becoming a better negotiator. He had near-perfect book knowledge of the subject. Yet when he engaged in an actual negotiation, he held back from applying all he knew because of feeling uncomfortable in performing his role. From this experience, he learned that he had to prepare himself psychologically before he could negotiate well. As a result, he now knows how to competently apply the discipline.

Having had one such application experience, many people would then believe that they had mastered the discipline. Wrong again! Instead, they have just gotten over the threshold of knowing how to apply the discipline. They won't begin to develop sufficient skill for mastery until they make enough more applications so that doing so requires little conscious focus on the required steps. In other words, they need to become unconsciously competent. After that, they will be able to resume applying the discipline whenever they want, even if a long time has passed between applications. When they resume applications, the experience will feel much like getting on a bicycle again after having once learned how to ride well.

Keep this explanation about mastering a discipline in mind when determining what you want to learn. Mastery may require many multiples of the time required for learning how to apply the discipline. Unless you will routinely face situations that will provide opportunities to apply the discipline, such time spent on mastery will necessarily come out of the time that you would normally devote to other purposes.

Enough said about mastery. Let's focus again on applying a discipline. Given that you have just learned how to apply a discipline, you may not yet appreciate what you should seek to accomplish when doing so.

I often see confusion about choosing an appropriate application in people who are learning how to develop 2,000 percent solutions (ways of being more than 20 times more productive with the same or fewer resources and time). Such people can typically recite all of the relevant steps, describe the caveats about what to avoid doing during the process, and talk knowledgeably about the questions that need to be answered. Yet very few of them will be able to define a specific goal for making some activity 20 times more productive. Instead, I will hear about intentions to "get faster at …" or "do better at …." When I push a little and ask that they describe what each of those statements means, I often receive some equally nebulous response. I've even had students who could never define a 2,000 percent solution goal with enough precision that anyone would understand what they were trying to accomplish.

What's my point? Well, it makes a great deal of sense to ask someone who has mastered the discipline to help you plan your first application. In doing so, hopefully the master will pick a subject

Lesson Five: Apply the Discipline

that's interesting to you. If not, push back until you can find an application that does appeal. Otherwise, you could easily lose heart during any difficult tasks.

Here's another consideration in picking an application: Which one will teach you the most about the discipline? For instance, some potential applications are going to arise much more frequently than others. If you first engage in one of the more common applications, you will have developed some expertise that you will be able to use more often. However, other applications might require using more elements of the discipline, potentially providing much more experience than would be gained by doing several other applications that required applying fewer of the discipline's methods.

In addition, you may well benefit from having a master help you select which aspects of the discipline fit your planned application. I often see this problem arising with students who are applying algebra and geometry to practical problems. If the assignment is in a textbook with narrow parameters tied to a chapter and section that explicitly describe what's being studied, then accurate solutions soon appear. If, however, the problem appears in isolation from such a chapter, in many cases the student might as well be addressing an impossible problem, due to being unable to think of any math techniques to apply in this situation.

If you become aware that you have difficulty knowing what aspects of a discipline apply to various kinds of problems, situations, and circumstances, I encourage you to do enough work in making such selections to master this skill. After doing so, you will then be able to select the most appropriate materials to refresh your memory about how to apply the correct aspects.

Finally, if the results of your work cannot be checked independently through some practical test, then you would do well to ask a master to review your work before determining that you have performed a successful application of the discipline. If you do not, you might have made quite a large error and have inadvertently "taught" yourself to make the same error during any future applications.

If you went to all this trouble to learn and then to actually apply a discipline, you must have had some good purpose in mind when you began learning. After completing such an application, review that purpose in light of your experiences to obtain a sense of its continuing relevance. Naturally, if the purpose was close to your heart and also to your calling for serving the Lord, the purpose is probably still appropriate. However, based on your experience and continuing prayers for the Holy Spirit to lead you to do God's will, you may well have developed a more specific sense of how best to use the discipline to achieve His purposes. If so, now is a good time to refine your plans for what to do next.

I can cite a personal example that may help. I felt called by God from quite a young age to study at a certain law school. With His help, I was able to fulfill that calling. While there, I certainly learned about the discipline. During my second year, I began applying what I learned by volunteering at a local community law office where I served people who could not afford an attorney. Because I did so on Saturdays, there was no one else in the office. I had to apply what I learned without any help. Through this experience, I realized that I would need to specialize and do much practice before I would become good enough at doing so. Although I liked the idea of helping the people, I was disappointed to find the actual experience made me feel very uncomfortable. Carrying the emotional burden of helping them felt too heavy for me.

After my second year, I then worked in a prominent law firm as a summer intern. This experience gave me a sense of what business lawyers do. I found this experience to feel even more uncomfortable. In fact, by 2 p.m. every day I developed a headache from doing the work. I couldn't wait for this job to end.

During my third year of law school, I reassessed my purpose for learning law and concluded that I should continue to apply the analytical perspectives, but mostly to do so for topics other than legal ones. I also decided I would handle my own legal affairs when I was qualified to do so. I went on to pass the bar examination so I would

Lesson Five: Apply the Discipline

be able to represent myself in any future situations requiring legal expertise. I also accepted a job as a management consultant where I found the kind of open-minded analysis I learned in law school to be quite helpful. I have found those choices about applying the legal training to be satisfying ones, ones that have enabled me to be fruitful in many ways that I believe God intended.

Having chosen these ways of applying my law school training, I then needed to focus my attention on learning and applying flexible, analytical ways of thinking that included more perspectives. Keeping that point in mind has been very helpful to me and made me much more fruitful for God's Kingdom. However, notice that I did not need to keep up on very many developments in the law, so my updating activities have been quite limited in that dimension of this discipline.

Similarly, you need to see how best to apply the discipline in the future so that you seek out relevant opportunities, stay up-to-date where important changes are occurring, and increase your skill in making applications. By taking time to make such an assessment after you first apply a discipline, you can potentially increase by many times the fruitfulness of applying your learning. Where possible, I suggest you look for ways to jointly apply what you have learned from several disciplines, as Peter Drucker did, so that you can become even more effective by drawing on more perspectives.

Your Assignments

1. What first application of your new knowledge about a discipline will be most useful in building your knowledge and skill in light of your initial interest in the discipline and how useful the experience will probably be?

2. Who can help you assess the relevance of such a first application for these purposes?

3. Who can help you decide how to best make such an application?

4. Who can review your results to correctly assess your effectiveness?

5. What did you learn from this application about how you should engage in applying the discipline in the future?

Lesson Six:

Teach Others and Keep Updating Information and Knowledge

*I beseech you therefore, brethren, by the mercies of God,
that you present your bodies a living sacrifice, holy,
acceptable to God, which is your reasonable service.
And do not be conformed to this world,
but be transformed by the renewing of your mind,
that you may prove what is that
good and acceptable and perfect will of God.*

— Romans 12:1-2 (NKJV)

Before CDs were invented, most recorded music was played on vinyl discs by using a needle to follow a spiral sound groove as the disc rotated on a turntable. Due to this physical contact, the sound quality from a disc was best when first used. After playing the same disc many times, the groove would wear and the sound wouldn't be as good. If you accidentally pushed the arm that held the needle sideways, you could actually cut a slash across the disc. If that slash was deep enough, your needle would then jump from where it was supposed to be on the recorded groove onto the slash before eventually

Lesson Six: Teach Others and Keep Updating Information and Knowledge

reaching a different section of the groove, thus skipping part of the recording. After enough play, you knew you needed another disc.

In a similar way, your effectiveness in applying a discipline can decline with repetition. Making mistakes is one reason that your effectiveness can drop. The first time you make a specific mistake, you may not notice it. If you also don't notice making the same mistake during subsequent applications, you might eventually develop a habit of repeating that mistake. As new mistakes pile up and are repeated, you could add still more erroneous habits, further reducing effectiveness.

Another problem arises from becoming overconfident. You may begin to take shortcuts, ones that cause you to make mistakes that you don't realize you've made. With more and more shortcuts, you can eventually become quite haphazard in your approach.

Romans 12:1-2 (NKJV) is a great instruction for all learners in this regard. We need to renew our minds before we will be able to do the good, acceptable, and perfect will of God. In spiritual matters, such renewal is done in a variety of ways including prayer, Bible reading, noticing circumstances, considering what's going on around us from God's perspective, spending time with other believers in spiritual studies, listening to the Holy Spirit, repenting sins, and asking for forgiveness.

As learners of secular subjects, we similarly need renewal. Reviewing what we've learned can help. Having others critique what we do while applying the discipline is another way to renew. Updating our learning and knowledge is still another way. However, in this lesson, I would like to focus your attention on the renewal possibilities that are best provided by teaching others. I do so because you may not otherwise engage in this important way to become and remain more fruitful.

My teaching experiences began when my sixth-grade teacher, Mrs. Gale, asked me to instruct my classmates in math. Part of her motivation was probably to keep me occupied so I wouldn't distract others. However, I also think she was a little impressed by my ability to rapidly solve problems. Most Fridays, I defeated my classmates in speed drills done on the blackboard. When I did, I took away the tasty treat of some candy as a prize, and I grew to look forward to those yummy bites of chocolate and almonds. My now-favorite ice cream is mocha almond, which reminds me of enjoying my sixth-grade treats.

During this teaching, I was quite surprised to realize that I often solved problems differently from how other students did. Almost all of them began at the beginning (the upper-left-hand part of a problem or page) and then proceeded through the material from left to right, and from top to bottom. My approach was more like that of a hunter: Find vulnerability and exploit it. I would, instead, view the whole material at one time. While doing so, I would look for a place to attack that would simplify and speed the task. I would then start from that place. My subconscious mind would then quickly leap to the answer. However, telling people to do the same as I did was of no help to them. Instead, they needed to see all of the steps to go through in a methodical way. So I again became a learner, this time deciphering and then articulating the steps I had unconsciously taken. The process was quite revealing to me. I learned more than my fellow students did.

In high school, I worked on my homework with a friend who found math to be more difficult than I did. By this time, I thought I knew how to explain processes. However, I found that my explanations often left her more confused than before I spoke. That's because I was explaining the process I used, rather than one she found understandable. From this experience, I learned to first comprehend how she thought before attempting to craft an explanation. Only those explanations that made sense to her mind were worth mentioning. Of course, I sometimes made mistakes in doing problems. When that happened, I was fascinated to see how her careful, step-by-step approach enabled her to spot all the mistakes I made ... most of which I was blissfully unaware of making. My learning continued on that front, as well. I began to appreciate the value of methodically checking from different perspectives.

Lesson Six: Teach Others and Keep Updating Information and Knowledge

Law school provided another chapter in my learning through teaching. I initially studied alone, while most other students shared their questions and ideas with one another. From studying, I learned the value of creating a good outline of each subject to review before tests. However, it was tiring and time-consuming to do so for all subjects. That's when I discovered that some students were willing to trade outlines. Of course, they only wanted to trade if my outline was a good one. Consequently, I learned to write better outlines. I also began to appreciate that others esteemed my taxation outlines much more highly than my property outlines. I began to ask about who was good at outlining what other subjects. I traded for those outlines. As a result, I was teaching others through my outlines, and they were teaching me with theirs. From this experience, I learned how to teach those I never met, an important step toward my future role in writing books and articles at God's direction.

After coauthoring *The 2,000 Percent Solution* (AMACOM, 1999), I was delighted to provide a course for graduate students to develop and apply 2,000 percent solutions. The first thing I noticed was that the book seemed to confuse students more than it helped them to apply the learning. They could tell me all the details of each step, but they could not perform all the tasks. I soon realized they needed something more like a cookbook, containing instructions on what to do that were broken down into simple chunks, something you know I highly recommend. The result, *The 2,000 Percent Solution Workbook* (iUniverse, 2005), enabled students to produce marvelous solutions, ones that were far better than I could have done. And the best part was that they needed little help from me while doing so. At the same time, I found I could also create 2,000 percent solutions with less time and effort.

The next pleasant surprise came when a student in that course proposed developing two related solutions that would multiply the benefits from each one. His intent was to increase revenues by 20 times while also reducing unit costs by 20 times. His work became the first application of complementary 2,000 percent solutions, ones that are described in *The 2,000 Percent Squared Solution* (Mitchell and Company Press, 2007) by Carol Coles and me.

Since then, I've been experimenting with in-person tutoring of students who want to master a variety of tasks. In doing so, I have learned many important lessons. First, I can quickly diagnose why a student is slow or makes errors by measuring those occasions and then discussing with the student how he or she went about solving a problem or answering a question. With a few more questions, I can discover what the student doesn't know, misunderstands, or hasn't considered. Then, in a few minutes, I can point out what needs to change and show many effective ways to do so. Some students make enormous improvements after just an hour or two of such discussions. Even those who don't learn as quickly can usually improve at more than 20 times the typical rate. For instance, writing students normally improve by three to four grade levels within a few weeks.

I also learned from such teaching experiences that many textbooks are poorly designed for rapid, effective learning and creating mastery. I was further convinced of this need and impressed by the potential value of taking a better approach while supervising one of my Ph.D. students while he prepared a physics textbook explaining better ways to apply math to identify where oil and gas might be found.

Have I stopped learning by teaching? No! I now frequently teach students who have been diagnosed with various learning disabilities. While doing so, I have gained many insights into how to refocus someone from engaging in a harmful activity over which she or he has little control into acting on a useful one. Many of these new lessons apply to all students.

Will God teach me more? You bet! But I'll have to keep teaching to gain parts of that learning.

From these experiences, I've also come to appreciate that I need to learn about subjects that had never previously crossed my mind. For instance, a recent discovery is that some students best learn how to solve problems by first learning how to design similar problems. I

Lesson Six: Teach Others and Keep Updating Information and Knowledge

now include such an approach for many curricula. In doing so, I've had to learn a good deal about how to design good problems. I suspect I will be learning lessons in this regard until my time on Earth ends.

Naturally, if I am going to teach someone a discipline, I also need to know the latest about that discipline. So I'm keeping up-to-date on more disciplines than before. As I do, new possibilities for breakthrough solutions occur to me. Methods in some disciplines, for instance, would be much more valuable for making breakthroughs in other disciplines than they are for the ones to which they are usually applied.

So what should you do? I'm going to defer most of that answer to Part Three: Teach Others, which contains 12 lessons for learning through teaching. However, keep in mind for now that you will learn more if you teach in a variety of ways. Each one will show you something you need to learn. As Part Three's lesson topics suggest, you will be helping students develop learning goals and understand how to apply a discipline's approach, testing learners for necessary skills, demonstrating multiple ways for them to learn any missing skills, drilling learners in those skills and tracking their progress, leading learners to adjust their skill-developing methods, demonstrating application of the discipline to the learner's goals, watching and correcting the learner's applications of the discipline, measuring and addressing the underlying causes of any errors, directing learners to self-improve the application process they just used, demonstrating appropriate ways to update information and knowledge, and then repeating the steps to teach still others. As you act in these ways, I strongly urge you to repeat your experiences with disciplines and skills that are newer to you so that you'll have more opportunities to be usefully stretched by your teaching. If doing so seems daunting, remember that you only need to be one lesson ahead of the students to be effective. So keep learning by teaching!

In Part Two, we expand on these first six lessons to give you greater understanding of how to effectively teach yourself.

Your Assignments

1. How can what you have learned by teaching yourself be made useful to new learners?

2. Where can you find such learners?

3. What should you do differently in helping them from what you did in teaching yourself?

4. How can their learning be accelerated?

5. How can they gain mastery in faster and more effective ways?

Part Two:

Teach Yourself

You, therefore, who teach another, do you not teach yourself?

— Romans 2:21 (NKJV)

In Romans 2:21 (NKJV), the Apostle Paul challenged those who knew and taught the Mosaic Law to others to act in accordance with that knowledge and such teachings. By contrast, when I was growing up, some teachers characterized how to learn from them as follows: "Do as I say, not as I do." Of course, that direction is just the opposite of what Paul advocated. What good is information and knowledge if we cannot accurately apply it to our own lives? Clearly, the matter is of great spiritual significance whenever something is done that opposes God's will.

In this part of *Breakthrough Learning*, you take on a significant challenge: Teach yourself to become a master of applying any discipline you wish. While you might not think that such a result is always possible, please realize that you should get help in a variety of effective ways while you learn. In addition, you might be concerned that you don't have as much skill as you need. That's okay. You'll be picking goals that fit with the benefits you want to gain, in light of the skills you have and can reasonably expect to develop or access through others. So think of this self-teaching task as a custom-sized one, one that perfectly fits you. After all, God made you into exactly the person He needs you to be to fulfill His purposes.

Part Two: Teach Yourself

Here's a preview of the nine lessons in this part. In Lesson Seven, you will learn how to find descriptions of the discipline's approaches and ways that they have been applied. You might already feel daunted by reading the description of this lesson. Relax! Realize that your search for disciplines will take you to places and people you aren't thinking about now, many of which will make the task much easier.

Let me share an example to help reduce your concerns. Imagine that you want to improve the income of struggling small farms that are owned and operated by poorly educated people. In doing so, you might first think that only advanced agricultural disciplines would help. What do you know about agriculture? Perhaps little, but God could still be calling on and using you to serve Him by improving these lives. Let's say that you then looked around, this time thinking about this issue as a business problem, rather than as an agricultural one. If you had contacted me for ideas in this regard, I would have told you that the discipline of developing improved business models is much more relevant than agriculture for making a significant improvement for such farmers. That's because simple business-model adjustments can cut distribution costs by 50 percent *and* raise revenues by 50 percent, while also substantially reducing the prices that consumers pay. Learning how to do so would take most people very little time. So when the research on this subject is broad enough to reach the sufficiently helpful sources, simple, easy-to-understand solutions are almost always available.

Much like this example, you'll be searching far and wide for appropriate disciplines to apply. In many cases, you'll end up just doing something elementary in a more effective discipline, rather than trying to push the state-of-the-art in some discipline that's difficult for you to grasp. Lesson Seven will show you how to make such searches, as well as relate where to find descriptions of applying the disciplines that you find to be relevant. You will also be encouraged, where appropriate, to engage with a discipline's masters to gain their insights into the approaches that should be used.

In Lesson Eight, we turn to determining the skills required to engage in a discipline's most effective approaches. Those who regularly apply a discipline are well aware of what practices they need to follow and what skills are required for engaging in those practices. As a newcomer to a discipline, you may lack such understanding. Here's another place where you may find it useful to contact experts in the field to find out what skills they and others regularly apply. If you cannot personally develop those skills, you'll need to find ways to access and apply the skills of those who already have such capabilities.

We focus next, in Lesson Nine, on setting goals for applying a discipline, a significant step for narrowing down what you need to learn to just what's necessary for the most relevant aspects of the application. Since you may not have done such goal setting, you'll be happy to find plenty of direction in this lesson to help you do so.

Lesson Ten then looks at developing the right types and levels of skills to implement the goals described in Lesson Nine. As we discussed in Lesson Three, it will be important to divide what needs to be learned into chunks of information and knowledge that can be easily understood and applied. You will learn more about how to do so here.

Next, in Lesson Eleven, we consider another task that requires proceeding in chunks: learning an effective process. In this lesson, I'll develop examples of what a process is, drawing on both the Bible and my own experiences. Then, I'll relate those examples to how you can logically proceed to learn a process.

Lesson Twelve helps you gain a more objective view of how well you are applying the process you've just learned. You will first identify ways to measure the performance of the process as you've applied it. After that, we'll look at the benefits of having your work checked. I'll also suggest how to find the right individuals to evaluate how well you've applied the process.

In Lesson Thirteen, you will find encouragement and directions to improve the process you just applied. Having read that description, you might be thinking that I'm asking you to operate as more than being an expert, to act as someone who can do more than what many experts can achieve: Make a better process. Instead, you'll find making such process improvements to be simpler and more valuable than you probably now appreciate. So, suspend any disbelief until you see what I propose here. Part of what makes this improvement simpler than you may think is that you will be designing a process that requires fewer skills, lower levels of skills, and less experience to perform effectively. Another reason why this redesign can be easy is that few practitioners may have taken any time to consider how advances in methods and applications might be combined for the first time to make a much more effective process.

Lesson Fourteen returns to the subject of updating information and knowledge. This time we look more closely at how a discipline's attributes, approaches, and processes determine what needs to be updated and how often. Again, we'll use a real example to make the advice more practical.

Finally, we'll take up the benefits of teaching others for advancing your learning and how to subsequently become aware of relevant new information and knowledge concerning what you learned through your teaching. In doing so, I'll continue with the example found in Lesson Fourteen.

Now, it's time to consider the topic of Lesson Seven: Find Descriptions of the Discipline's Approaches.

Lesson Seven:

Find Descriptions of the Discipline's Approaches

Then he said to me,
"The north chambers and the south chambers,
which are opposite the separating courtyard,
are the holy chambers where the priests
who approach the LORD *shall eat the most holy offerings.*
There they shall lay the most holy offerings —
the grain offering, the sin offering, and the trespass offering —
for the place is holy.
When the priests enter them,
they shall not go out of the holy chamber into the outer court;
but there they shall leave their garments
in which they minister, for they are holy.
They shall put on other garments;
then they may approach that which is for the people."

— Ezekiel 42:13-14 (NKJV)

You may recall from the Introduction that a discipline is often the same as an academic field of study, such as art history or mathematics. A discipline can also be narrower, such as applying mathematics to determine how much accuracy a sample of information brings for answering a question, a discipline called statistics. Beyond that, eval-

Lesson Seven: Find Descriptions of the Discipline's Approaches

uating certain types of samples in applying statistics could present particular challenges, ones that will require specialized applications that will, in turn, constitute a still narrower discipline. And on and on specialization goes into narrower and narrower applications.

Chances are that you won't know the identity of all the broader and narrower versions of a discipline when you begin. However, you should assume that identifying and learning about them is part of your task in finding descriptions of their approaches, the topic of this lesson.

In doing so, you may find Ezekiel 42:13-14 (NKJV) to be a helpful source of instruction. In these verses, the prophet Ezekiel described what a man in a vision showed him about how the priests should place and eat the most holy offerings and choose their garments depending on whether they were in a holy place or just with other people. In describing what garments priests should wear, these verses capture the Godly view of priests, as well as the ordinary perceptions of people who aren't priests. You can see that such a small point about something as apparently unimportant as what should be worn can be significant to God, a good example of why it's important to accurately understand how a discipline works best.

From God's perspective, the Holy Spirit can direct you to just the disciplines and descriptions needed for you to begin learning. God is, as you know, all-wise and all-powerful. So be sure to go to Him seeking directions. In doing so, God might guide you to look in certain places or to ask specific individuals. Immediately do what He says. In other cases, God may send people to you, much as He sent Ananias in Acts 9 (NKJV) to take away the blindness that Paul experienced while meeting Jesus on the road to Damascus. If you don't find such Godly directions leading you to where you need to go or other people to you, assume that God is presenting you with a test that will, instead, develop you spiritually, such as by helping you to become more patient.

If you are to do much or all of this seeking of descriptions on your own, start by looking into basic sources, the kind that are used to teach a discipline to newcomers. Such sources might be included in a syllabus for an introductory high school or college course. If you cannot locate such sources, reference librarians are among the most underutilized and valuable resources for such purposes. If your request is a simple one to answer, they'll work on it while you wait. In other cases, there may be a slight charge to do a more thorough search on their own time. If you happen to live in a community (as I do in the Boston area) where there are many universities, you may find that there are specialized libraries at such schools focused on just the disciplines that initially interest you. Reference librarians in these libraries may be able to tell you off the top of their heads where to look. If you don't happen to live in such a place, you can always do online research to locate a highly regarded disciplinary library and call a reference librarian there to ask for help.

What if you don't know what disciplines to look into? For instance, the study of black holes involves astronomy, as well as theoretical physics. While you might imagine that you needed to know about astronomy, theoretical physics might not occur to you, especially if you've never studied the subject. In such cases, you would be helped by finding a book about black holes and checking the backgrounds of the authors, as well as those of the text and article writers cited by the authors. In doing so, you'll find many clues. If you are stuck at this point, you could always contact one of the book's authors to ask which disciplines would enable you to appropriately study the subject. Naturally, if you know more specifically what you want to learn, explaining that interest may well enable the author to direct you even more appropriately to the correct disciplines.

In many cases, today's graduate-school students are more aware of the cutting-edge practices of a discipline than are even some renowned authors and professors. Many of the best students provide tutoring to those who want to learn a subject. You could find such a knowledgeable tutor and ask for help in finding the right disciplines for your learning interest, as well as for finding out how those disciplines' approaches are conducted.

Lesson Seven: Find Descriptions of the Discipline's Approaches

As you do such seeking, I suggest that you also ask about any other disciplines that might provide valuable insights. For instance, most disciplines would be greatly improved by more often conducting online contests that provide significant opportunities to gain reputation or practical benefits for having identified enhancements. Consequently, learning how to design and implement such contests could be quite relevant to any discipline that you study.

Another way to identify valuable disciplines is by scanning for instances where large improvements have recently occurred that affected people who are somewhat similar to those you intend to serve. You can also ask those you contact about successful examples of improvement that have impressed them. From investigating such examples, you will sometimes locate relevant disciplines that you should also understand.

Let's assume now that you've found several disciplines that are relevant. Simply because I've referred to finding descriptions of a discipline's approaches, you could be assuming that experts usually write books and articles on that topic. If you are assuming that, I've misled you and I apologize. In many cases, you would look long and hard to find even one of such writings. What you would find, instead, are many descriptions in books or articles of how someone conducted research (or experiments) and analytical activities in a discipline that led to important new learning. When you find one such description of recently discovered knowledge, you will sometimes be able to decipher what is being said to appreciate how the discipline was applied in this instance. After you read several of such descriptions, you'll probably develop some hypotheses about how the discipline goes about improving information and advancing knowledge. At that point, you will benefit from discussing what you have concluded with someone who regularly applies the discipline. As you do, work from the perspectives contained in the assignment questions found in Lesson One.

As you find or develop these descriptions of approaches employed by a discipline, I encourage you to think about how easy or difficult each one will be for you and others to apply. I make that point because in many cases you will have a choice of disciplines, and choosing the ones that are easily applied will potentially speed or even multiply the benefits that are gained. However, don't reject a discipline that presents difficulties that you can learn to handle but which also provides vastly more potential benefits.

For example, The 400 Year Project has three broad approaches that can be applied for making breakthroughs: 2,000 percent solutions, complementary 2,000 percent solutions (where each such solution also increases the benefits of each other solution by another 20 times), and excellent solutions (providing the same benefit as from 10 complementary 2,000 percent solutions by developing only one solution and making just one set of changes). While these disciplines range from least difficult (2,000 percent solutions) to most difficult (excellent solutions), the differences in benefits are far greater than are the differences in difficulty. As a result, someone who wants to accomplish the most should apply excellent solutions. With but just a few of such solutions, the ways that almost everyone lives would be dramatically improved.

In fact, these three 400 Year Project approaches are so close to being universal in application that at least one of the three is surely appropriate for some aspect of what you want to accomplish. So if you don't find any other disciplines that seem directly related to achieving a great deal, be sure to include one or more of these three approaches.

Once you have found promising disciplines and appreciate their approaches through studying how they have been applied, you will be ready to think about how to apply an approach to what interests you. In doing so, I cannot urge you too strongly to find experts to discuss how each discipline might be applied to your interest. If you sense that you may want to combine approaches from more than one discipline, be prepared to explain your idea in enough detail so

Lesson Seven: Find Descriptions of the Discipline's Approaches

that single-discipline experts can react to what you propose. To do so, you may have to briefly introduce them to the approaches of one or more other disciplines so that the expert can intelligently consider the feasibility of what you are considering. For instance, if you are going to combine two or more disciplines, the concerns of both experts should help you see where bridging any gaps between disciplines and their approaches might be required. Naturally, if you can find an expert who knows both disciplines and their approaches, such a person's reactions will be still more valuable.

Even if God has sent you off to find the proper disciplines and approaches on your own, don't forget to check your understanding with Him before completing work on the tasks involved in this lesson. Doing so will help you to be more humble, while also to stay on the right track.

Your Assignments

1. What has God revealed to you about which disciplines and approaches to apply?

2. Who is in a position to help you find descriptions of disciplines and their approaches that fit well with what you want to accomplish?

3. How can you access these individuals?

4. What do you want each of them to do?

5. What resources can you use to increase access to them?

6. After finding or developing descriptions of disciplines and their approaches, who can test your understanding of those descriptions?

7. Who can test your thoughts about which approaches to apply?

8. Who can check your understanding of how to apply what seems to be the ideal approach?

9. Who can evaluate your understanding of how to apply approaches from more than one discipline?

Lesson Eight:

Determine What Skills Are Required

*And Moses said to the children of Israel,
"See, the* LORD *has called by name Bezalel the son of Uri,
the son of Hur, of the tribe of Judah; and
He has filled him with the Spirit of God,
in wisdom and understanding, in knowledge and
all manner of workmanship, to design artistic works,
to work in gold and silver and bronze,
in cutting jewels for setting, in carving wood, and
to work in all manner of artistic workmanship.
And He has put in his heart the ability to teach, in* him
*and Aholiab the son of Ahisamach, of the tribe of Dan.
He has filled them with skill to do all manner of work
of the engraver and the designer and the tapestry maker,
in blue, purple, and scarlet* thread,
*and fine linen, and of the weaver —
those who do every work and those who design artistic works.*

— Exodus 35:30-35 (NKJV)

When we do a task for God, naturally we want to apply as much skill as possible, aided by the Holy Spirit while doing so. We find a helpful reminder about the importance of having the right skills and

Lesson Eight: Determine What Skills Are Required

how to find them in Moses' description of who should do some of the work to produce the Tabernacle, where God was worshiped during most of the years while the Israelites were living outside the Promised Land after escaping Egypt. You'll notice in this case that Bezalel and Aholiab were amazingly gifted, having abilities for creating and implementing artistic designs with the finest craftsmanship. Bezalel is further described as having wisdom and understanding, consequences of being filled with God's Spirit.

As I mention in Lesson Seven, you are likely to find more descriptions of how a given discipline has been applied to solve a specific problem than you are to find general explanations of how the discipline works. For the purposes of this lesson, this difference in availability is an advantage. While reading about an application of the discipline, you can imagine yourself and those you know engaging in the activities that are described. As you so imagine, make note of any skill and knowledge requirements that you don't yet have.

If you are unaware of how to learn what's required, you should research the subject by looking into the training engaged in by those who do such tasks professionally. Once having identified such a profession, chances are good that you can also find someone who works in that profession. After having done so, you can ask such an individual about the methods and how any difficulties of gaining the knowledge and learning the skill compare to the challenges and costs of hiring people to effectively apply their good knowledge and skill.

Of course, if the descriptions of applying the discipline are far beyond what you can understand, you'll need to speak with an expert who can answer your questions in simple ways about what knowledge and skills are necessary, how to acquire them, and alternatively how to access such knowledge and skills through volunteers or hiring able people.

I'm sympathetic to this problem of being lost while trying to understand what's required. I was 12 years old when I first became interested in space exploration. Wanting to grasp everything I could, I was pleased to see a book at the library about selecting trajectories and speeds for putting satellites in orbit. However, I was baffled by what the book contained. I couldn't even follow the math through what was in the first chapter. Of course, the main problem was that I had not yet progressed beyond pre-algebra. So the mathematical expressions in the text were alien to me. At the time, the experience made me feel more like someone who didn't have a future in doing calculations relevant to space exploration than like someone who did. Had I known to ask someone about acquiring the necessary skills to do such calculations, I probably would have been told that in due course I would be able to handle the work just fine. Had I known that likelihood, I suspect I would have taken more advanced math classes in college in hopes of ultimately being able to apply what I learned to space exploration in some useful way.

Let me provide a few special cautions about appreciating what skills are necessary and how to acquire them. First, descriptions of applying a discipline's approach will often emphasize certain aspects of the work, while totally ignoring others. For instance, if the work involved in applying the approach is substantial enough that it needs to be done by a large team, then someone is going to have to be good at recruiting and managing the members of that team. A description of the work is highly unlikely to mention either of such tasks. Instead, you might pick up the idea from scattered references to finding the right people and of getting the work done in a cooperative, timely way.

Second, for projects that were reasonably expensive to do, someone had to pay the bills before the time when any benefit accrued. Most descriptions of applying a discipline will omit any reference to the work involved in obtaining such funding. If you have never sought money to pay for an expensive application of a discipline's approach, it would be easy for you to underestimate what is involved. I know that I once assumed that any good purpose could find funding. With more experience under my belt, I now appreciate that there are many more attractive-sounding uses for money and resources than there are funds and people to supply all such uses.

Lesson Eight: Determine What Skills Are Required

That's one reason why I always emphasize engaging in tasks that require very little, if any, additional funding and resources. For instance, The 400 Year Project (see Appendix B for an overview of developing three fundamental approaches for accelerating the rate of global improvements by 20 times) was funded almost totally by donations of volunteer time. The volunteers (me included) supplied from our own resources almost all of what little was needed in terms of facilities, equipment, and cash.

Third, the power of many findings to be influential can be greatly multiplied by a powerful analogy, metaphor, or demonstration. For instance, some people didn't pay much attention to Einstein's early work on gravity affecting light until measurements during a solar eclipse validated his theories. The results were front-page news, something that doesn't occur very often for spreading new information and knowledge. By contrast, the publication of my work on business-model innovation occurred on the very day when the world was waiting to see what would happen when U.S. troops first entered Baghdad during the second Iraq war. Not surprisingly, there was little interest that day in the results of this kind of organizational innovation. Consequently, valuable information was left dormant by many people simply due to this shift in their attention. Attracting interest in the right way can be one of the most difficult skills to learn for accomplishing certain applications of disciplines, especially for those that require widespread usage to be effective.

Let me shift over now to considering how else you might determine what skills are required. One method I've found to be quite helpful is to "shadow" someone performing a task. Here's what I mean. Rather than only gaining intellectual knowledge of how an approach is implemented, you can observe someone doing an approach. If the agreement to follow the person is a cordial one, you'll also be able to ask questions about why the individual does what she or he does. The answers will often amaze you by their candor and helpfulness. That's because in the heat of doing something, those with the appropriate skills and experience have the easiest time appreciating what might be relevant for someone else to learn.

Of course, there's an even more effective method: Participate as part of a team that has all the needed skills. However, since you are undoubtedly going to be quite inexperienced and potentially may lack some of the relevant skills, such teams may often be reluctant to let you participate in this way. In your younger years, you can often participate as an intern, a way to see what's going on, to do some useful things, and not have anyone mind if you slow matters down a bit from time to time.

Let me share a personal example to explain how joining a team can help. When I first worked as a management consultant, I had only taken two business courses in my life, both relating to marketing. Yet, I was now supposed to offer strategic advice to CEOs of major companies. How could I do that?

I learned how to do such consulting by traveling with officers of the consulting firm as they did their work. What I discovered was that they could relate a series of stories about business experiences (what were then called "war" stories) that captured the attention of senior executives concerning strategy. In addition, the officers had presentation materials that introduced strategic concepts that most CEOs thought were fascinating. Within weeks I learned to tell the same stories and present the same materials. Of course, I also mastered answers to the kinds of questions that were most often raised by CEOs. Within three months, our firm's CEO was flying me off to meet with CEOs and other senior executives of large companies on my own. It worked just fine, even though I looked as if I should still be in high school. From then on, I was able to do what I recently had no idea of how to do. It was a fascinating experience. I hope that you will have many like it.

If you can't learn the skill on your own, relax. The good news is, of course, that the world is filled with people who have superb skills, even the rarest and most valuable ones. As a result, I've rarely run into a situation where it was impossible to either learn a new skill or

Lesson Eight: Determine What Skills Are Required

to attract sufficient help in an affordable way to accomplish an important application of a discipline. So stick with it!

Your Assignments

1. What skills do you perceive were necessary to employ the approaches you found in reading about how to apply this discipline?

2. How are those skills different from those that were necessary for related approaches in other disciplines?

3. What skills might be required that are not explicitly stated in the descriptions of the approaches?

4. Who would know exactly what kinds and levels of skills are necessary?

5. Who would let you shadow him or her while she or he conducts such an approach?

6. How could you become part of a team that is employing one of these approaches?

Lesson Nine:

Set Goals for Application

*And we know that all things work together for good
to those who love God,
to those who are the called according to* His *purpose.*

— Romans 8:28 (NKJV)

Romans 8:28 (NKJV) is one of those verses that you can meditate on for a lifetime and not fully appreciate all of its implications. One of the hardest lessons for most people to learn from this verse is that God can generate good results from even their worst mistakes. An even harder lesson is that God can create good results from the bad things that evil people do. While those who think of God as being all-powerful and all-knowing can often intellectually appreciate such points, such possibilities can seem more like having head knowledge about a fictional story than feeling like a reality-based belief. Thus, those with only head knowledge may not act with full faith in God's unerring ability to bring good out of anything, even intense and apparently unwarranted suffering. I was reminded of this lesson in yesterday's sermon at church, as the pastor shared two testimonies of long and apparently unnecessary suffering that the sufferers came to see as blessings by helping them to draw closer in their relationships to Jesus through better understanding His sufferings for us.

Lesson Nine: Set Goals for Application

There can even be problems for someone who does have deep and comprehensive knowledge of and experiences with God's goodness. Since God can do it all, some who believe in His abundant abilities might conclude that there's no point in setting the right goals. Let me politely differ with this view. While God certainly doesn't want us to worry about anything, He does have a purpose for having us set goals: He wants the goals to clarify for us and others whether we are doing our best to serve His purposes. In the course of doing so, God gives us this task as a way to purify our hearts so that we can have a better relationship with Him. After all, think about what it would be like to daily review a set of goals for engaging in some important work for advancing God's Kingdom. Surely, focusing on these goals would help align your heart and mind more closely with Him.

In addition, appropriate goals help us to notice when we or others are straying from where He wants us to place our attention. While focused on Godly goals, we are also less likely to be distracted by the lusts of the flesh, the lusts of the eyes, or the pride of life.

If you agree that goal-setting is an important part of building your relationship with Jesus, please continue reading this lesson. If you are still in doubt about the wisdom of doing so, I suggest you use key word searches of the Bible to help you find verses that will bring you peace about what God is calling you to do in this regard. Also, pray for guidance about what God wants you to do.

When I think about what a goal is, I immediately imagine looking at a basketball hoop, the metal ring from which a net hangs. If you put the ball through the hoop from top to bottom, your team earns one to three points, depending on the circumstances under which your shot was taken. If the shot is a "free throw" after being fouled, each ball through the goal is worth one point. If a shot is made from the court while time is running and the other team is contending, two points are earned. If the ball is launched under the same circumstances while the shooter's two feet are behind the arc painted on the floor beyond the free-throw line, three points are counted.

If you've ever played basketball or even just watched a game, you know that the ball takes up a pretty high percentage of the space within the hoop. Hit that rim in the wrong way, even with the ball mostly being on target for the goal, and the ball can fly far from the goal. So it's a pretty precise thing to score a goal in basketball.

I think that the goals for applying your learning need to be similarly precise and closely related to the nature of the effort you intend to make. Otherwise, you, too, might have a near-miss that actually sends the results of your efforts careening far from where you intended.

I always encourage people who are setting goals to start with what kinds of benefits they would like to create or increase. While the answer might seem simple in the abstract, in practice choosing a proper benefit can be far from obvious or easy. Let's imagine that you want to eliminate poverty in a certain community. How does such a desire translate into a benefit? Is it to raise the income of the person, improve some aspect of the person's quality of life, increase the person's ability to take care of her or his own needs, or decrease the person's use of resources? Picking the right benefit goal in such a case might mean first doing some research to understand what the effects of such changes are, as well as how those effects relate back to reducing poverty. As you can imagine, the answers are often far from clear. And if you prayed for guidance about such a question, you might find that God directed you, instead, to focus on poverty of the spirit, something that affects even those who are materially well off.

Let's assume that you've found a useful benefit to provide. What, then, should be your goal for how much of that benefit to make available? Once again, some research might be necessary. What kinds of results are obtained when people apply the disciplines and approaches that you favor? How many resources are you likely to have for the purpose of producing these benefits? How long will it take you to become effective? And so on. By contrast, realize that God can multiply the fruitfulness of your efforts through attracting others to work with you, as well as by potentially making supernatural provisions. Naturally, you'll want to know how God wants you to think about the size of what you should accomplish. For instance, in my case God directed me to find ways to accelerate the improvement of each and every aspect of human activity, from the mundane to the spiritual, by more than 20 times. As my experience demonstrates, He can send some pretty big orders. When that happens, He undoubtedly wants to build your faith.

Although I mentioned the idea of eliminating poverty in a community, there's still the question of whose poverty. For instance, in a household that contains at least parents and children, the household might meet the definition of not being a "poor" one in a material sense, but some members of the household might be living with too few resources. For example, imagine that a parent needs a heart transplant. Until such an operation occurs, this parent is certainly going to be poor in terms of health.

Timing is important for setting most goals. For instance, if God had told me to meet His goal for advancing the rate of improvements by 20 times after only an hour had passed, I could have done virtually nothing in this regard without His supernatural support. However, He graciously granted me 20 years to demonstrate and document how to do the work, while the Holy Spirit often whispered what to do in my ear. The next goal He directed me to accomplish was for such a speed-up in improvements to occur globally by 2035. We've still got a ways to go before the deadline, and I'm quite interested to see how He will enable this goal to happen. I make that comment because although what to do is already well documented, few people are doing so. That's because most people prefer to do things in the much less effective ways that they already understand. In terms of your goals, I encourage you to pick a time to start and consider having goals for what is to be accomplished over different time periods along the way, as God did with me.

Let's say that you are having trouble setting these kinds of goals. Again, pray for His guidance. If He doesn't answer specifically, ask

Him where to seek help. He may direct you toward an individual, a source, or even to an experience that will enlighten you. If you don't receive such directions, you can still find many people on your own who have had good experiences with setting goals. You probably know some of them already. Ask people who share your heart for what you want to accomplish to suggest people with skill in goal setting and check out those individuals.

Of course, if the learning goal only affects you, you naturally need to focus on how well it will clarify your direction and keep you encouraged. However, in many cases your learning goal will affect many other people. In such instances after you develop goals, you also need to check to see if the goals are understandable to people who didn't participate in setting them. Speak with a few of each type of stakeholder (all those who are affected by what you will be doing or accomplishing through achieving the goals, such as beneficiaries, family members of beneficiaries, those who will take actions to generate the benefits, people who will provide needed resources, and those who will supply any needed knowledge or skills). As you can imagine, if such stakeholders are confused by the goals, harm can ensue; even in the best case, time, effort, and resources will be wasted.

Having spoken with many people who have had good success with goal setting, I'm struck by how many of them describe how encapsulating the goal into an empowering story can make a positive difference. For instance, I find that many capable people don't want to delegate very much of what they do to others, correctly appreciating that they can do the tasks better than many other people can. In taking this approach, such individuals often forget to consider what could be accomplished if they, instead, spent their time in more productive ways. The story I tell in this regard is about a CFO who had once supervised every element of company's annual budgeting process, spending more than 100 working days each year in doing so. Then, he decided to delegate the task to another staffer. Doing so reduced the CFO's time involvement from 100 days to only 3 days. He then applied the 97 days to working, instead, on ways to improve company profits, and the results were counted in the tens of millions of dollars annually. Additionally, this CFO's relationships with the other executives improved, since he wasn't the one asking pointed questions about proposed budgets. Few people who hear that story fail to start delegating time-consuming tasks.

Creating understanding is one thing; creating enthusiasm is another. If the goals and stories have inspirational qualities, more people will be attracted to help and will provide more assistance while doing so. Here's a story one of my students shared with me. He was invited to speak at an economic development conference held on an island populated by about two million people. Speakers described how valuable it would be to create more jobs, but no one mentioned any way to do so. After the conference, my student decided to stay on for a few days, touring the island. Along the way, he saw what facilities existed, what kinds of skills the people had, and what the land could grow. He promised to return in a few weeks, this time bringing with him experts in agriculture, tourism, and small-scale manufacturing. Drawing on what these experts recommended, goals were set to upgrade tourist facilities, shift agriculture to higher value crops, and start producing hand-made goods made in beautiful local designs. To turn the goals into reality, my student shared these opportunities with caring entrepreneurs he knew who then helped to either set up new businesses to make such changes or to help the local people do so. Within a short period of time, the island's economy was experiencing a fine expansion for the first time in many years. My student's passion and his empowering descriptions of the possibilities had made all the difference between people simply wanting to do more ... and taking appropriate actions that worked well for meeting the goal.

Your Assignments

1. What results are needed to be most fruitful?

2. What goals can accurately capture what needs to be done for whom?

3. What is an appropriate timeframe for steps in the goals?

4. Are those goals understandable to stakeholders?

5. Do those goals inspire stakeholders to take action?

6. What stories related to the goals can improve understanding and inspire stakeholders?

Lesson Ten:

Develop Types and Levels of Skills for Application in Chunks

And let our people also learn
to maintain good works,
to meet urgent needs,
that they may not be unfruitful.

— Titus 3:14 (NKJV)

As Titus 3:14 (NKJV) reminds us, being fruitful for God by doing good works and meeting urgent needs is one useful way of applying our learning. Hopefully, your goals include such an application. If not, consider if you should make any adjustments to your goals.

If the skill-identification work described in Lesson Eight and the goal setting described in Lesson Nine have been done correctly, you are now ready to develop the necessary skills to meet your goals. Keep Lesson Three in mind as you do, being sure to appropriately narrow down what is to be learned into appropriate chunks of information and knowledge so that understanding and application can occur more rapidly and effectively.

During this lesson, keep in mind that while developing such information and knowledge obviously applies to you, all of those who

Lesson Ten: Develop Types and Levels of Skills for Application in Chunks

will be involved in the application will also need to learn. Even if some of those who will be engaged are quite expert in what they do, all of them will at least need to gain information about and understanding of your goals and how their expertise and efforts should fit with whatever else is happening.

To divide information and knowledge into easy-to-learn chunks, I suggest that you keep in mind that many people primarily learn by visualizing what's involved, conversing about a subject, or having a related, revealing experience. While it's tempting to just focus on the one of these three learning manners that you prefer, you will find that anyone will learn more through using all three of these methods. While each of us has a favorite method, we are all capable of gaining much more useful information and knowledge by being engaged in all three ways. The more impact each of the methods has, the better the combination of them will work.

Finding ways to be exposed to or to provide simultaneous visual, auditory, and physical experiences requires breaking down what is to be learned into chunks that permit such an approach. Let me use a simple example to make this approach clearer.

Let's imagine that you want to learn how to use a hammer to attach two pieces of wood with a narrow-headed (often called a "finish" or "finishing") nail. Let's assume you have no experience with hammering such nails. For the first chunk, you might arrange to watch a video about how to select the right kind and length of nail (it's good for one to have a head with a dimple in it to hold the nail set and to be of a length 25 percent shorter than the depth of the wood to be nailed), hammer (flat-headed), and nail set (containing punches whose tips are smaller than the head of the finishing nail) for the purpose. Then you might go to a home center or hardware store to discuss any purchases of nails, hammer, and nail set with someone who has experience in high-quality carpentry. After having this discussion and obtaining all the necessary supplies, you could watch a video that directed you in ways to practice the steps involved. Such a video might begin by demonstrating where the nail should be placed. You would then practice doing so with someone who would instruct you and comment on your effectiveness as you did so. After you had mastered where to place the nail, you might watch a video about how to start hammering a nail. This action typically involves gently tapping with a hammer while holding the nail between the thumb and forefinger of the other hand until the nail is firmly inserted a little way into the wood at the correct angle. After watching the video, you would have someone demonstrate doing so, observe you doing the actions, and comment on how well you performed them. For the final chunk, you would be instructed in the same manner (by using a video, in-person demonstration, commentary, and feedback) for learning how to perform the remaining steps (hammering the nail's head without striking the wood until it is just above the wood's surface, and then tapping the punch while its tip is in the nail's dimple to lower the nail head to just below the wood's surface). From there, learning would focus on the correct ways to practice, repeating any needed demonstrations, and regularly reviewing and discussing observed performance.

When you wanted to learn how to teach someone else to hammer narrow-headed nails, you would repeat what I've just described by taking on the role of the person who provides instructions for what to do, demonstrates performing the proper practices, and provides feedback on how well those practices have been performed by the learner. In this instance, you would also need someone to observe your work with the learner and give you feedback on how you could improve in directing the learner. Such observations of your teaching would continue until such time as your observer and you were confident that you understood what to do. The observer would then advise you in how to develop and maintain teaching mastery. In the future, you would occasionally have someone observe and comment on what you were doing. Naturally, in all circumstances where you help others to learn, you should also ask learners to provide ideas for how you could improve.

Lesson Ten: Develop Types and Levels of Skills for Application in Chunks

Let's translate this nail-driving example into how the learning process might be more generally applied. Keep in mind that for each chunk you would combine visual, conversational, and experiential elements in as close conjunction as possible.

Begin by defining one or more chunks for becoming oriented to what will be required. Before being able to design the orientation, you would probably first have to spend time observing how someone does what you want to learn. If you could also ask questions while the activity was being done, that would be even better. If you could try performing some of the tasks, that's even more desirable.

After such an introduction, you could start to become oriented. One chunk might be for preparing to learn, a chunk which might include setting an agenda for what should be accomplished before starting to learn, selecting the right environments for learning, and obtaining necessary resources, such as videos, tools, materials, and access to expertise. If the work involved is complex or difficult enough, each of these possible parts of preparing to learn could also become a separate chunk.

After conducting the orientation chunk or chunks, you would then focus on the first learning task related to developing the skill. In selecting this chunk, you might focus on a necessary first step. However, if one part of the learning will take much longer than other parts, or will affect the ability to do the other parts, you might choose to focus sooner on that particular learning aspect. For example, when I help students for whom English is not a native language prepare for standardized tests, I first work on their reading skills. I do so because all aspects of such tests require highly effective reading. After developing more of such skills, performance in all parts of the test improves. Consequently, the amount of work required for learners to become more effective in other elements of the test is greatly reduced. In some cases, the need for other learning from me may be entirely eliminated for those learners who are then able to effectively read and apply helpful learning materials on their own.

As you develop each chunk, think about how it can be designed to better integrate with the other chunks that follow. For instance, a chunk for developing reading skill might include written materials that will be needed during a later learning chunk.

Beyond that, if you need to develop more than one skill, consider how the content of chunks for the first skill might include valuable learning or exposures to information that will be applicable for gaining a different skill. Don't stop there! Look for ways to integrate material from all the skills you need to develop into the chunks for the other skills. Such early exposure and repetition will make you much more effective in accomplishing your learning goals.

Once all the skill-development learning tasks have been reduced to chunks, you would then accomplish the same thing for any experiences that are needed to improve any skills that are different from the ones in the initial learning. For example, you might focus first on a reading method that enabled effectively scanning more material as a learning chunk. To then gain experience in this reading method, you might have another learning chunk that included researching all relevant information in connection to any of the other learning experiences you will need.

Naturally, you'll also need learning chunks for teaching others what they need to know, even if they will only play the role of observing and commenting on your teaching methods. Of course, at the point when you are actually ready to begin teaching others to apply your new knowledge and skill, you'll need to develop further chunks for doing so. An initial chunk for such teaching might simply focus on identifying potential learners for you to instruct. We'll focus in more detail on teaching others in Lesson Fifteen.

Your Assignments

1. How can you spend time with those who are applying a skill you need to develop?

Lesson Ten: Develop Types and Levels of Skills for Application in Chunks

2. How can such experiences enable you to obtain answers to your questions about how to develop the skill?

3. How can these experiences also provide you with a hands-on feel for applying the skill?

4. What steps are needed to sufficiently develop one skill?

5. How can the order of the steps be used to increase your understanding?

6. How can such steps be broken down into chunks?

7. How can the content of one chunk provide an earlier appreciation for a later chunk?

8. How can the content of one chunk provide an opportunity to begin learning a different, but related, skill?

Lesson Eleven:

Learn and Apply an Effective Process in Chunks

*Now Isaiah had said,
"Let them take a lump of figs,
and apply* it *as a poultice on the boil,
and he shall recover."*

— Isaiah 38:21 (NKJV)

Chapter 38 of Isaiah (NKJV) contains an extremely interesting example of a process that God used to accomplish His purposes. Let me use the events of that chapter to introduce you to what I mean by a process.

At the chapter's beginning, King Hezekiah of Judah was "sick and near death." Isaiah was sent to relate to King Hezekiah what God had told him, "Set your house in order, for you shall die and not live."(Isaiah 38:1, NKJV)

Hezekiah didn't like what he heard. He turned his face to the wall and prayed to God, reminding Him of his faithful service. Hezekiah then wept bitterly. (Isaiah 38:2, NKJV)

God heard the prayer and responded by sending a new message for Hezekiah through Isaiah the prophet. The message was also validated by a promised sign. "Thus says the LORD, the God of David your father: 'I have heard your prayer, I have seen your tears; surely

Lesson Eleven: Learn and Apply an Effective Process in Chunks

I will add to your days fifteen years. I will deliver you and this city from the hand of the king of Assyria, and I will defend this city.' And this *is* the sign to you from the LORD, that the LORD will do this thing which He has spoken: 'Behold, I will bring the shadow on the sundial, which has gone down with the sun on the sundial of Ahaz, ten degrees backward.' So the sun returned ten degrees on the dial by which it had gone down." (Isaiah 38:4, NKJV)

It was only after the second message was delivered by the prophet to King Hezekiah that Isaiah issued the very ordinary sounding instructions for what medical treatment to apply, to place a simple poultice of figs on a boil.

In the normal course of events, we wouldn't expect that placing some figs on a boil would extend the life of a sick person who was near death by even a little while, let alone 15 years. God may have appreciated that Hezekiah would be skeptical of His answer to his prayer. While He could have provided evidence of His promise in a variety of ways, including healing Hezekiah so quickly and completely that he immediately leapt out of bed and danced around the room, God, instead, chose to provide one of His most remarkable demonstrations: occasioning this sundial's shadow to proceed backwards, rather than forwards, by ten degrees. As the verse describes what happened, the sun seems to have moved backwards in the sky by ten degrees before returning to its regular pathway from east to west. Isn't that amazing?

Let's now break down what happened in this chapter into a process. I'll do so by describing the pieces of the process as different, sequential steps.

As the verses open, Hezekiah had already fallen gravely ill. That condition triggered the need for a process. For accomplishing your learning, you will have already set goals to change something about existing conditions.

Think about how extraordinary the purpose was behind God's first step in this process: choosing to send a message of impending death. My impression is that most people don't receive any messages from God that are delivered by a famous prophet just before they die. While we do not know from the Bible what God's purposes were in doing so, it's possible that He just wanted to hear from Hezekiah. Another possibility is that God wanted Hezekiah to act in a certain way, possibly including the selection of a new king, so that the succession after his death would be smooth and lead to the proper person. Notice that God allowed plenty of room for free will, such that Hezekiah could take either a better or worse action in response to the announcement.

The second step was to send the message for Hezekiah to Isaiah. We aren't told how this was done.

The third step, of course, was Isaiah presenting the message to Hezekiah. If Isaiah hadn't known where to find the king or needed to be introduced to him, there would have been some intermediate steps required before the message could have been delivered. Since God can speak to each of us personally, I have always wondered why God did it this way. Perhaps He had already tried to get Hezekiah's attention through the Holy Spirit, and the king had ignored or misunderstood the message.

The fourth step was Hezekiah deciding to pray for God's help. Notice that this step extended the process into more steps. Otherwise, Hezekiah would just have died as God had announced, and his death would have been the final step in the process. This fourth step should always remind us that God likes us to draw closer to Him, and He's prepared to respond when we do.

The fifth step was Hezekiah's actual prayer, one in which he reminded God of his faithfulness in serving Him. We see several examples in the Old Testament of successfully bargaining with God by those who presented valid arguments to explain how God's Kingdom would benefit more by His taking a different action than a just-announced one. We should always be prepared to do the same with God. In addition, we should work with others connected to a process to be sure that they are aware of how their actions can advance

God's and their own interests in better ways than what would occur with the originally intended actions.

The sixth step was God's consideration of the prayer. While God didn't reveal His thought processes in these verses, such a consideration probably preceded His decision. After all, He was next going to change Hezekiah's fate in a way that was different from what He had just communicated. Otherwise, this revised decision would not have reflected God's perfect intent.

The seventh step was God deciding what He wanted to do. Undoubtedly, the expression of Hezekiah's heartfelt plea was part of what influenced God to develop other choices for accomplishing His purposes, ones that would demonstrate how great His power is. Choosing to extend Hezekiah's life when he was so ill would certainly make such an impression. To top that, God indicated He would defend Jerusalem against and deliver it from the enemy that had plagued Judah for so long. But those wonderful promises were just warm ups for the *pièce de résistance*: causing the sun's shadow to move backward. Regardless of how God caused the shadow to move backward, the effect had to be very impressive to observers, as well for all of us who can only read about it and be amazed. God surely knew this sign would be a compelling exhibition of His unlimited, righteous power that would stand for all time.

The eighth step was God communicating his second message to Isaiah. Again, we are not told how this occurred. The message could have been sent through an angelic messenger, the Holy Spirit, some sign, or in some way beyond my imagining.

The ninth step was Isaiah presenting God's second message to Hezekiah.

The tenth and subsequent steps involved God acting to fulfill each of His promises: extending Hezekiah's life, defending and delivering Jerusalem from the invaders, and causing the sundial's shadow to move backward by 10 degrees. When those actions were done, the process was complete. God's purposes were accomplished.

Breakthrough Learning

What God did to cause each of those three results might have also entailed other process steps, such as directing an angel to do certain things. However, these details aren't revealed in the Bible. I don't want to speculate on these methods, so I'll stop this example here. I hope you now better appreciate how steps can split a process into the elements that must occur before a proper result can be accomplished.

Just in case this example didn't help you as much as you would like, perhaps a simpler example could be useful. When you walk up a flight of stairs, you move from one stair step to a higher stair step. Each time you do, you have taken another process step required for you to reach the top of the flight of stairs. I also hope this example helps.

Let's focus now on why processes are important. As a youngster, I didn't appreciate the potential value of following the right process until I began assembling plastic pieces to produce model airplanes, ships, and cars. The instructions for doing so always seemed to be printed on the flimsiest possible paper and in type so small you almost needed a microscope to read them. There were also hard-to-decipher diagrams and really boring steps to do. Does anyone really want to check each part in the box to be sure they are all there before doing anything else?

When I first made such models, they had relatively few parts, the parts were fairly large, gluing them together wasn't very tricky, the decals were easy to handle, and painting was pretty simple to do. So I could just start putting things together any old way. I just assumed that all of the parts were present, and my assumption was correct.

Later, I began to assemble extremely difficult models with large numbers of teeny parts, delicate decals in very small sizes, and directions for adding microscopic bits of paint in many different places. The first time I did so, I proceeded as usual by putting things together in the order that appealed to me, rather than by following the instructions. Within 13 minutes, I had made a mess of that model, a mess that I couldn't completely clean up. Since the model had cost

Lesson Eleven: Learn and Apply an Effective Process in Chunks

me the equivalent of three days' wages, I was quite upset. After that, I never again tried to assemble a model without rigorously following the directions ... as best I could understand them, which often wasn't very well.

Similarly, if we do the right steps in the wrong order, the results won't be the same. Imagine if God had started the process by moving the shadow back on the sundial. Would Hezekiah have responded then in the same way when Isaiah told him that he would soon die? Imagine if Isaiah had directed that the poultice of figs be put on Hezekiah's boil without Hezekiah first having issued his prayer. Would Hezekiah have been healed? I'm sure you can see my point: In a process where one step opens up helpful possibilities for what can happen next, you need to proceed so that those possibilities are open before acting on them. Otherwise, the result might be like what would happen if a man first observed a woman who appealed to him and then immediately walked over to propose marriage. She wouldn't take him seriously. If he had, instead, first developed a good relationship with her over a long period of time, the proposal might have been received more favorably, possibly even welcomed.

Let's not forget about chunks. While process steps might appear to be chunks, performing the necessary steps might require further breaking down what's involved in a step. Here's an example. I'm getting ready to visit three countries in Africa later this year where I will be sharing ways to expand and improve God's Kingdom. To do such sharing, I'll need to prepare differently for each set of people I will meet. So while doing such sharing would be a step in a process, there might be quite a few earlier chunks involved, such as my first finding out what these people want to learn, what they already know, what information will be mostly helpful to them, and how they can most effectively appreciate what is shared. If, as in one case, they want a PowerPoint presentation, learning how to do so in a way that would be most effective for them will involve quite a few chunks for me. I intend to ask audience members to send me examples of PowerPoint materials that they have found to be most effective. If available, I could benefit from studying videos of the presenters of such materials. In addition, I will prepare a draft of the presentation and have the person who is most concerned about the relevance of my presentation review it with me and make suggestions for improvements. And I could repeat these chunks after I did each revision of the presentation materials.

So, take each step in the process and break it down into chunks that represent useful ways to accomplish the step. Be sure to sequence those chunks in the most effective order, as putting them in an incorrect order can potentially be as harmful as putting the process steps in the wrong order. If you have any questions about how to do any of such ordering in a particular instance, feel free to contact me by e-mail at donmitchell@fastforward400.com so that I can help you.

Your Assignments

1. What are the steps in the process you intend to apply?

2. What aspects of these steps do you need to learn?

3. Who can teach you to effectively perform such steps?

4. Do you need to break the learning for how to do such steps into chunks because either different people will need to teach you or the focus involved needs to be narrower?

5. What orderings of those steps can cause problems?

6. What orderings of the chunks for a step can cause problems?

Lesson Twelve:

Measure Performance and Have Your Work Checked

*But let each one examine his own work, and
then he will have rejoicing in himself alone, and not in another.*

— Galatians 6:5 (NKJV)

Examining your own work in a fair and honest way can be hard to do well. After all, you made many of the decisions about what to do without the influence of anyone else. Surely, you liked those ways of doing things or you wouldn't have chosen them. In addition, it can be hard to separate the positive and negative effects of unexpected shifts in circumstances from any effects of useful actions or mistakes you made. Also, the sources of some effects may be hard to uncover.

I find two things to be extremely humbling: comparing myself to God *and* looking at all the mistakes I've just made. Each humbling influence works in a different way, squeezing my foolish pride concerning what I've done to the subatomic size that it deserves to be, much like the way a powerful vise can compress a piece of balsa wood. However, no matter how humble I feel, I'm still incapable of spotting all of my mistakes. Why? Well, I have this difficulty, in part, because I make too many mistakes while looking for my mistakes. Now, isn't that ironic? So I think of the verse in Galatians 6:5

Lesson Twelve: Measure Performance and Have Your Work Checked

(NKJV) as just the starting point for finding out by how much my work needs to be improved. For instance, I certainly wouldn't want you to read this book unless it had already been thoroughly gone over by an outstanding editor, my long-time guide to writing better books, Bernice Pettinato.

What solutions for evaluating work would be effective for you (as well as for me)? Begin by measuring outcomes. Hopefully, your application of a process was accompanied by setting an expectation about the results your work should accomplish. If the process didn't set such expectations, you may still be able to measure what at least some of the results have been.

Consider that many of the most effective processes also contain ways of measuring effectiveness during steps, so that adjustments can be made before errors cause much harm. For instance, when I had cataract surgery, the receptionist asked me which eye was being operated on that day. After checking her records to see if my answer was the same, she put a band on the wrist for that side of my body. When I met the first nurse, she asked me the same thing, checking that the wrist band was in the right place. After that, the anesthesiologist asked me the same question before pumping me full of Valium and whatever else left me in a dreamy state. Then, on the operating table, the surgeon asked me which eye was to receive treatment. At that point, I felt quite confident that the correct eye was going to be operated on before the surgeon cut into me.

The finest processes (especially for those that have the potential to cause great harm) typically have backup steps prepared for dealing with failures that could affect any essential elements. For instance, if a valve in the life-support system on a manned space vehicle gets stuck, there's usually a way to make a manual adjustment. Doing so is much like having a plumber stop a leak under your sink, except in this case an astronaut might have to personally wield the wrench.

If the process you are following does not include such backup preparations, then you can use continually measuring whether every aspect is working properly (as the surgical-center staff did for having the correct eye be operated on during my cataract surgery) to avoid harmful errors. If your process doesn't already have such measurement steps, make some notes about what's needed. You'll want to think about ways to overcome such limitations during the process-improvement work that's described in Lesson Thirteen.

If you are like me, sometimes just measuring the results of a step or the whole process may not sufficiently identify the source of a problem. Imagine that I want to bake a cake. I might follow all the directions to a "T" and still end up with a cake that's soggy in the middle, despite having seemed to be done when I poked a toothpick into it. I could probably think about that problem for quite a long time and not come up with all the likely answers. However, an expert would probably be able to put her or his finger on the source without much thought. Chances are that the issue relates to something about the oven I used. Perhaps the electric-heating elements weren't working uniformly, so that the edges of the cake received much more heat than the middle. If I happened to stick my toothpick closer to a well-done edge than to the middle, I might not realize that part of the middle was still soggy. After cutting into the cake and discovering the problem, there's little that can be done except throw the middle away. The oven would have to be fixed before adequate results could be achieved for another cake. Despite this risk, I've never seen a cake-baking recipe that included instructions for first checking whether the heating elements of an electric oven were properly functioning.

In contrast, sometimes you can get perfectly acceptable results without realizing that an error had been made, due to the mistake having been offset by an unperceived, favorable circumstance. For instance, when I push the "pizza" button on my microwave to heat up a slice, 60 seconds of power are applied. However, if I have a large piece of pizza, it will still be cold at the end of that time. If I warm up the large piece for another 60 seconds, then it will usually be fine. Yet the effect of doing so isn't the same as heating the same slice of pizza for 120 seconds, because there has been a cooling off

Lesson Twelve: Measure Performance and Have Your Work Checked

period between the two occasions of 60-second heating. Also, if the piece of pizza is much smaller than a large one, it doesn't need as much heating time. I'll only discover these relationships after I heat a small slice for 120 seconds and end up with shriveled brown cheese and dry tomato sauce on cooked dough that resembles burnt toast. I know that's true because that's the result I created when I heated my small piece of pizza for lunch today.

My recommendation is that you decide how to check your performance before you apply a process for the first time, adding measurements to as many points as possible that would indicate if a problem is about to occur. For instance, if I had taken my small piece of pizza out when I first heard the cheese bubbling, it would have been fine. However, despite hearing that sound, I stupidly let the microwave continue doing its thing without considering what was probably happening inside. I also could have watched through the window in the microwave door, noticed that too much browning was starting to occur, and stopped the microwave at that point. Shame on me for ignoring my own advice!

If more than one person will be engaged in performing the process, be sure that measurements capture exactly what is done. Otherwise, you could be comparing someone's faulty memory or false impressions of *what was* done to what *should have been* done. I see such misleading comparisons occur all the time with students. After having a problem applying what they've been studying, they *always* tell me that they have *perfectly* followed the directions. However, when I ask them to describe how they did so, they leave out many of the important elements. If they write down what they just did at each step, I can gain a pretty good indication of what was actually done ... unless, of course, the person purposely writes something false.

If more than one person will be affected by the process, you may find that measurements will need to be customized to reflect the circumstances of each individual. For example, someone who assembles a product will be affected differently than many of the people who use the same product. Consequently, a different set of measurements is needed for understanding the effects on the assembler than for the effects on the users.

Naturally, you will be using such measurements to avoid errors, as well as to identify how the results of steps vary from what you expected. While doing so, pay even more attention to overperformance than to underperformance. Why? Overperformance may reveal potential ways to make breakthroughs, while any underperformance will only tell you about mistakes and conditions that you should have been paying attention to (such as the size of the pizza slice in my example).

With many good measurements in place, you may be wondering why you would need someone else to check your work in applying the process. Let me explain about my experience last week in checking the work of a student team that was preparing a business plan for a new product. The measurements for the effectiveness of this plan included regular reviews by the rest of the team as well as weekly comments from the professor concerning the work to date. However, the team had failed to appreciate many of the fundamental issues involved with implementing the plan. Why didn't these reviews overcome that problem? Well, the plan was so vaguely written that the reviews mostly focused on requesting more specifics. Then, the next draft of the plan would also be produced with too little detail. As a result, the underlying issues remained hidden. As the outside observer in this case, I was able to point out what some of those hidden issues could be. No one else perceived them. Without that timely review from an objective source, the final plan would have been a disaster.

Another problem with your own reviews can be that you may have insufficient experience to realize what the information means. Here's an example of that problem occurring during my long-ago work as a new development director. I had just toured a retail store that had made an astonishing sales improvement. I knew that I had identified something important. However, there were no records to help me see what had been improved that might have caused the re-

Lesson Twelve: Measure Performance and Have Your Work Checked

sults, and the person responsible wasn't available. The on-site employees simply said that the new leader had done a better job of following procedures. While I didn't appreciate it at the time, this information was an important clue to the reason why many of the business problems experienced at other stores occurred: not following procedures, mostly due to ineffective leadership and poor training. Eventually, these causes were identified as being pervasive and were effectively addressed. However, due to my lack of experience, I missed an opportunity to get the ball rolling several years earlier. Had I been joined by someone with more experience who had a more objective perspective, the proper inference might have been drawn on the spot.

Having now gained a sense of the potential value of having your work checked, there's still the issue of finding the right individuals to do so. Someone with long experience in applying the process in the same ways as you are doing should be able to do a good job. However, if the individual isn't very good at applying the process, you might not learn as much as you could from someone who has more expertise. I suggest you ask several individuals with the necessary skill and experience to do so.

I saw the benefit of multiple perspectives recently demonstrated while planning for some repairs in our home. The original builder propped the floors of two lower-level rooms atop wooden posts placed directly on the ground beneath. Since the wood hadn't been pressure-treated and the ground wasn't isolated from moisture, the wood had become wet and started to rot. As the weight above the floors compressed the rotting posts, the floors began to sink. Two structural engineers told us at different times that the problem lay with our cement slab sinking due to the ground beneath it being eroded. Well, there was no cement slab under these rooms; the engineers had been too lax to look beneath the floors to see what was happening. So much for their "expertise" doing us any good!

Then, we had a number of contractors look at the problem and propose solutions. One of them eventually noticed the actual source of the problem. We told the other contractors so that we didn't get any more recommendations to raise the "concrete slab." However, rarely did any two of the contractors agree on what needed to be done. Based on our experience, we didn't think structural engineers were going to give us good answers for sorting out these views. So we had to find people who had already solved such a problem and obtain their views of the potential solutions. Naturally, we didn't want to rely on just one point of view for doing so. After gaining such advice, we were finally able to select a good method.

Your Assignments

1. What are the outputs you seek to gain from applying the process?

2. How can you measure those outputs in terms of how they affect each person?

3. Where can measurements help you avoid making costly and harmful mistakes during the process?

4. What should these measurements be?

5. How should those measurements be used?

6. Who should evaluate how well you have performed the process?

Lesson Thirteen:

Improve the Process

"If you take away the yoke from your midst,
The pointing of the finger, and speaking wickedness,
If you extend your soul to the hungry
And satisfy the afflicted soul,
Then your light shall dawn in the darkness,
And your darkness shall be as the noonday.
The LORD will guide you continually,
And satisfy your soul in drought,
And strengthen your bones;
You shall be like a watered garden,
And like a spring of water, whose waters do not fail.
Those from among you
Shall build the old waste places;
You shall raise up the foundations of many generations;
And you shall be called the Repairer of the Breach,
The Restorer of Streets to Dwell In."

— Isaiah 58:9-12 (NKJV)

When something important is first done, there is often a scramble to meet a deadline, come in under budget, or cope with a severe limitation that seems immovable. During all that turmoil, however, there will be fleeting quiet moments during which those involved might think, "Surely, there's a better way." Because of a sincere desire to

Lesson Thirteen: Improve the Process

do the right thing during the first applications of a process, most people will be cautious, strictly following whatever the experts suggest. However, the existing process could have been developed before many of today's alternatives and much of our current knowledge existed. Surely, such a process should be reevaluated after being experienced for the possibility of including what can be done now that wasn't possible before.

What if you can't think of any alternatives to the process, despite being displeased with the first experience? Humbly turn your heart and mind towards doing God's will and pray for guidance from the Holy Spirit. He will provide you with directions to improve the process. That's the clear promise of Isaiah 58:9-12 (NKJV) for those who have been faithfully serving God.

Also, take another look at all those examples you read about for applying the process while you were learning about it. Were there any variations in the methods used? Is it likely that any of the variations you didn't apply could have produced better, faster, or less expensive results for you? Could any of those variations be substituted for elements of or be used as supplements to the process you employed?

Some processes proceed slowly because they require the assistance of highly skilled people who may not be immediately available when needed. Reviewing the process just used may suggest ways to supply more information and directions for what to do so that those with less skill and experience can operate as, or even more, effectively than highly skilled individuals who lack such support. When such a substitution of personnel can be made, then the work will usually proceed faster and less expensively. Due to not having as much experience, such individuals can sometimes bring open-minded questions to the tasks that improve the quality of the ultimate solution.

Here's an example of making such a successful substitution for less expensive personnel. A property-casualty insurer learned that it was spending more time and money than it could afford to process small damage claims. One of my students found the process to be needlessly complicated and time-wasting for people who could contribute more by doing other work. She realized that over 80 percent of the process steps could be eliminated if those who were physically closest to the damage could do the initial claim processing locally and then transmit their work electronically to the home office. Then there would only need to be a final review by one person to ensure that the procedures had been correctly followed before paying the claim. Providing information, knowledge, and directions to the local people enabled this change, eliminating over 95 percent of the small-claim-processing costs and reducing the length of time before a claim was paid by over 98 percent. An unexpected benefit was that the company gained market share by adding desirable customers who were interested in having faster claim service.

The people who conduct a process and are affected by it can also be helpful sources of improvement ideas. If the people performing the process feel that their time is being wasted, they will often use their underoccupied minds to think of ways the work could be made simpler, easier to accomplish, and more interesting. Of course, some of such doers may remain silent due to worries about retaliation from their colleagues who like the way the process is done now. If you make providing such suggestions safe to do, you'll soon have a number of useful ideas to pursue. Also consider that those who receive or benefit from the offering or service often have acute sensitivities that cause them to be clear about what they would like to have done differently. It usually takes little encouragement to gain the benefit of their sharing with you what they see as undesirable, wasteful, or unnecessary.

A key limitation of applying such advice is that most of the suggestions will point to only minor improvements. So be sure to take the time to sort through the suggestions to focus your attention and effort on those few areas (probably less than 5 percent of suggestions) that could provide over 80 percent of the value of potential improvements. If you do so, a significantly more effective process will undoubtedly emerge.

Lesson Thirteen: Improve the Process

Also, check for what any critics and reformers of the discipline have been saying about the weaknesses and challenges of employing your and similar processes. If you contact such individuals, they may be able to direct you to people who have experimented with making such changes. In addition, ask about as-yet-untested adjustments that critics and reformers feel should provide substantial improvements. Sometimes, making such an adjustment successfully can be as simple as applying the results of some excellent, related research that most practitioners are ignoring.

Another helpful method for finding improvements is to lay out the whole process as a flowchart on a big piece of paper or a white board. Leave room next to the steps in the flowchart for how the process is done now to write alternatives. Identify steps that add relatively little value and take too long. Can any of those steps be eliminated? If yes, do so. If that's not possible, look into how some of such steps might be combined so that delays or costs are reduced. Most processes involve nothing being done during over 95 percent of their durations. Reduce those idle moments, and the length of a process can be greatly shortened. For instance, while it normally takes many months to build a new home, the process can be greatly speeded up by making preparations in advance that enable moving promptly from one sequential task to the next. As an extreme example, for the purpose of setting speed records, homes have been totally built in just a few hours. Shelby County Habitat for Humanity accomplished such a feat on December 17, 2002, by constructing a fully functional house on an already prepared foundation in only 3 hours, 26 minutes, and 34 seconds.

Another source of delays can be having too many people rechecking what has already been checked. If you can find ways that error rates can be reduced by noticing and remedying mistakes as they occur, you can eliminate almost all of such checking and rechecking. For instance, in assembling an electronic product, you can have some of the most important testing be done by assemblers who have been trained to fix the usual sources of problems right there and then. Obviously, such an approach is easier to do if they work in an assembly area, rather than on an assembly line. Consider if such major adjustments in process methods might have other substantial benefits, such as Toyota found for increasing quality and reducing costs by shifting its vehicle production to assembly areas instead of using the American model of assembly lines.

Consider another source of delays that we have all experienced: waiting in line. Many banks, supermarkets, and mass merchandisers have separate lines for customers to be helped by each service person. If you happen to pick the wrong line, you might wait much longer than if you had selected one where transactions are conducted much faster. While having one customer queue for all the service people is an obvious improvement, you may be able do even better by letting people check themselves out ... or conduct transactions without anyone else being involved. In using such approaches, better-run organizations typically have one service person present in the vicinity for handling any problems. If what's required is easy, convenient, pleasant, and fast for customers, such a combined approach can be effective.

While I could go on to list a large number of potential process improvements, seeing this information might cause you to feel that you had to investigate them all. That's not the purpose of this lesson. Hopefully, these limited examples have given you a sense that there should be ways to substantially improve any process, especially if those who typically apply it haven't often tried to do so.

There's a side benefit to be gained from addressing this opportunity that might not otherwise have occurred to you. Perhaps you didn't fully understand the process when you first applied it. While looking for improvements, you might just locate something important that you were supposed to do that you somehow overlooked!

Lesson Thirteen: Improve the Process

Your Assignments

1. Where did you find the process to be ineffective, awkward, slow, expensive, or unnecessarily complicated during your first application of it?

2. What do those who were involved in applying the process think should be improved?

3. What do beneficiaries, end users, and customers dislike about the process?

4. What changes do those who were involved in or were affected by the process advocate?

5. When did delays occur because of needing to involve highly skilled people?

6. How can less skilled people perform more functions well after being provided with added information, knowledge, and directions?

7. How can steps be simplified, combined with other steps, or eliminated?

8. How can errors be caught and corrected sooner and with less expense?

9. How can other sources of delays be eliminated?

10. What new information, knowledge, or resources can be used to improve this process?

11. How can useful methods found in similar processes be applied to improve this process?

12. How have applications of this process sometimes differed in ways that should always be employed?

13. How can advance preparations speed the process, enable it to work better, or reduce its costs?

14. What else do you wish could be done faster, better, or less expensively during the process?

15. Who could help you identify other ways to make such improvements?

Lesson Fourteen:

Update Information and Knowledge — An Example

> *Then He who sat on the throne said,*
> *"Behold, I make all things new."*
> *And He said to me,*
> *"Write, for these words are true and faithful."*
>
> — Revelation 21:5 (NKJV)

In the book of Revelation, John describes a vision of what will happen in the end times. There will be a new heaven and a new Earth. All will be made perfect, not just new. In Revelation 21:5 (NKJV) that vision is summarized while underscoring the significance of this prophecy.

Similarly, we need to seek new information and knowledge as resources for coming closer to the heavenly perfection that God wants for us. Isn't it wonderful that He is providing for us in this way, even before replacing the current heaven and Earth?

Until such time as He delivers the prophesized perfection, we should be doing the best we can here on the old Earth. By now, however, you might be feeling a little weary of my references to updating information and knowledge. Hopefully, I can provide you

Lesson Fourteen: Update Information and Knowledge — An Example

with new insights in this lesson that will improve your understanding of such updating, as well as what's involved, by providing an example, one that continues in Lesson Fifteen.

One of the most visible, recent examples of the value in updating information and knowledge can be observed in the process that professional baseball teams use to search for better players. I have long been aware of this discipline and its processes because of first having applied statistics to evaluating baseball decisions as a youngster for a science-fair project. Since then, I have updated my information and knowledge in this regard on many occasions.

To introduce this example, let me describe the origins of this search process. Throughout much of the 20th century, professional teams gathered information about prospective players with a combination of having former players watch games as scouts and looking at a few key statistics, such as batting averages for hitters and earned-run averages for pitchers.

The first important improvement in these methods came in the 1960s when it became possible to measure the speed of pitches during a live game. Prior to that, pitching speed was simply estimated by scouts, often inaccurately. Obviously, a fast ball with more velocity is harder to hit. By being able to also measure differences in the speed of other pitches (such as change-ups, curves, and sliders) by that player, a better estimate of potential effectiveness could be obtained. In doing so, teams could appreciate what could be accomplished if pitchers used their talents optimally, something that did not often occur while inexperienced catchers were selecting pitches. Initially, how to best use this new information largely involved guesswork. After a time, teams learned how to use it better through considering how prior recordings of such information matched the later success of the same pitchers.

Prior to that time, television had already introduced the ability to create moving images of the pitch's path. However, for a variety of reasons, these images were inaccurate. Only after 2010 did some major-league teams start to locate cameras in places that provided more accurate depictions of what happened between the ball leaving the pitcher's hand and its passing home plate, the target for gaining a called strike from the umpire. Prior to that time, scouts and analysts could only estimate the movement of pitches by relying on misleading perspectives. If you sit in different locations in several ballparks, how a pitch looks will be greatly affected by the shift in perspective. Picking up the "movement" of a fast ball, for instance, is quite subjective without having accurate straight-on camera views. For instance, some players and commentators occasionally describe fast balls that "rise," something that good camera evidence demonstrates doesn't happen.

Technology wasn't the only reason that new information became available. Some fans were fascinated by the opportunity to measure more about what happened in games. By defining new ways that performance could be described by using existing measures, new forms of analysis could be applied. For instance, a new statistic was developed for estimating how much ground a fielder could effectively cover by comparing fielding results to what happened when others played the same position, rather than by just looking at whether successful individual catches and tags or throws were made.

Since the 1980s, statisticians have been producing many other analyses based on newly developed measurements that are more useful for evaluating a player's overall performance, whether as a pitcher, a hitter, or a fielder. While some teams became quite intrigued and began using these new statistics to make their player-selection decisions, others did not. Awareness of the results of such differences was greatly increased by *Moneyball* (W.W. Norton, 2003) by Michael Lewis, which describes the evolution of such measures and statistics, focusing on their use in player selection by Oakland Athletes general manager Billy Beane. While his team had far less money to spend for players than its competitors, the Athletics often won games more frequently than their spending levels suggested should occur. The book provides evidence these better results happened because other teams undervalued some forms of player performance, such as the

Lesson Fourteen: Update Information and Knowledge — An Example

ability of batters to gain walks or to get hits when runners are already on base.

Inspired by evidence that more and better information could improve team performance, technologists began working to find ways to more precisely measure what happens during the game. For instance, recent technology improvements have provided ways to measure a large number of aspects of how a player attempts to field a ball, such as how fast the fielder accelerates towards the ball, not just whether the attempt is successful or not (and whether the official scorer characterizes any poor results as an "error"). Naturally, all such measurements can be added to other useful ways of selecting players.

Where will these searches for better information and knowledge end? It is pretty clear that new and improved measurements and analyses are going to continue to advance knowledge of player performance. The result should be better decisions about which players to obtain and retain. In addition, much of the information could improve coaching by helping to identify ways a player needs to change. Managers should also be able to make better decisions about what players to put on the field or at bat in various situations.

As you can see, baseball has transitioned from employing a player-selection process that relied on the subjective credibility of former players into one that increasingly builds on objective, verifiable information that can be analyzed in a large number of ways. That's quite a big shift. Interestingly, it's a shift that has yet to occur in many other processes. For example, when I work with companies to understand how well they maintain and improve their most important processes, much of what I observe involves trial and error conducted by experienced people. In some cases, the processes are so dependent on the skills of a single individual that they cannot be maintained when that person is no longer available. Taking such an approach is a bit like trying to produce a great performance of a difficult aria without having an opera singer who can perform the role with requisite skill.

Let's consider what characteristics of updating information and knowledge about processes are most likely to be valuable. First, be sure you understand how objective or subjective a discipline's process measurements are. The more subjective such measurements are, the greater will be the potential to improve what is done by developing and applying more objective information. Also, be aware of the potential for measurements to be made still more objectively and accurately. Sometimes this potential is accomplished by making more measurements. In other cases, new methods or technology will be needed to enable enhancements. Use your appreciation of what information is missing to focus your attention on just what you most need to track. I also suggest that you look into similar fields to identify what is being done there. Doing so may give you advance understanding of what improvements are likely to come next. Finally, be sure that you directly consider the potential of any new or improved measurements to accomplish more.

Next, let us look at approaches for applying new information. While new data may be available due to new measurements being made, not everyone is going to use them. Such differences of opinion about what to apply can provide valuable insights into the value of new measurements. For instance, in a context such as baseball where competing methods affect relative performance of organizations or individuals, you may be able to analyze the impact of such different applications. In addition, you can speak with those who use various approaches to better understand why they chose one method rather than another. It may be that some of them would like to switch approaches, but are blocked by a disagreement with a superior. As an example of how this can occur, consider that those who don't understand much about statistics are less likely to see doing more of such analysis as a potential benefit. Be aware that subtle differences in approaches can often be valuable to consider. Always check to see if the factual context is influencing any of such differences. For instance, a baseball team without any good left-handed pitching may choose to use a different statistical approach for player selection as one that is well endowed in this regard.

Sometimes differences in approaches don't relate to information usage. Here's an example. Some approaches favor adding more training or practice before individuals begin using a process. Doing so may permit using a simpler process due to being able to rely on those employing the process to make more adjustments when needed. Another difference in approaches can be in how much is done for beneficiaries, customers, and end users. In many cases, you may find that doing less actually creates better results by permitting beneficiaries, customers, and end users to make more of the valuable adjustments they prefer than can be easily done on their behalf.

Processes will also continue to evolve, including the development of totally new processes that can replace some or all of what is done now. Sports often reveal this potential for developing new processes. Consider how high-jumping methods have become obsolete through several revolutions in just the last few decades. Adjustments to existing processes may, instead, relate to changing the sequencing of steps, or simply to adding or deleting steps. Again, be aware of any new versions of processes. As with approaches, be careful to understand how the context has affected such a process choice. Then, compare the context to your own to determine its relevance.

I also encourage you to look outside the perimeters of your discipline's attributes, approaches, and processes, such as for identifying substitutions and replacements. After all, the market for electrified streetcars is much smaller now than it was before World War II. Even though a substitute (a gasoline-fueled vehicle in this case) may be less fuel efficient, preferences of stakeholders may mean that a shift will occur anyway. In this case, people are more sensitive to privacy, comfort, and flexibility in route and timing than they are to the cost of transportation. When such preferences affect decisions, you need to be ready to operate effectively in terms what they are, rather than in optimizing what you've been focused on.

While I could provide many other potential sources of information and knowledge to consider, I'm sure you get the idea: Keep your eyes and ears open!

Your Assignments

1. What sources of information for conducting your process need improving?

2. How could such improvements be made?

3. How can you monitor such information improvements?

4. How can analyses for conducting your process be improved?

5. Where might some improvements occur?

6. How can you monitor such analytical improvements?

7. What other attributes of your process could be improved?

8. How can you monitor such attribute improvements being made by others?

9. How can approaches to your process be improved?

10. Where can you monitor such improvements in approaches?

11. How can your process's approach be improved by others?

12. How can you monitor such process improvements?

13. What substitutes or replacements for your process might be developed?

14. How can you monitor any such substitutions or replacements?

Lesson Fifteen:

Teach Others and Stay Up-to-Date — An Example

So Moses' father-in-law said to him,
"The thing that you do is not good.
Both you and these people who are with you
will surely wear yourselves out.
For this thing is too much for you;
you are not able to perform it by yourself.

Listen now to my voice;
I will give you counsel, and God will be with you:
Stand before God for the people,
so that you may bring the difficulties to God.

And you shall teach them the statutes and the laws,
and show them the way in which they must walk
and the work they must do.

Moreover you shall select from all the people able men,
such as fear God, men of truth, hating covetousness; and
place such over them to be rulers of thousands,
rulers of hundreds, rulers of fifties, and rulers of tens.

Lesson Fifteen: Teach Others and Stay Up-to-Date — An Example

*And let them judge the people at all times.
Then it will be that every great matter they shall bring to you,
but every small matter they themselves shall judge.
So it will be easier for you, for they will bear the burden with you.*

*If you do this thing, and God so commands you,
then you will be able to endure, and
all this people will also go to their place in peace."*

— Exodus 18:17-23 (NKJV)

Exodus 18:17-23 (NKJV) relates the sage advice of Moses' father-in-law, the Midianite priest Jethro: You need help with all the small stuff that's overwhelming you! This advice also applies to us today.

In the context of breakthrough learning, such advice has a special significance: After others learn what you know, you can accomplish even more by also observing and learning from the applications your students make. While applying the process, such learners will cover ground that you would never have time to consider. By keeping up-to-date on what your students do, you can then selectively extract important lessons that should be applied to your own work, thus greatly multiplying your effectiveness. If you and your students engage in making the same kinds of improvements, then the multiplied results (with God's grace) can be even greater than what you would be able to accomplish by yourselves.

Let's look at some of the limitations of relying solely on official sources of information and knowledge. Formal disciplines often encourage updating what is known in the field through publishing the best peer-reviewed new work in journals. By tracking such publications, you can stay informed about what the editors consider to be the best new information and knowledge. Of course, much of what is learned never appears on such pages. In some cases, that's true because there's a benefit to keeping a secret, such as for developing or maintaining a valuable advantage in some application. In other cases, a person who lacks strong sponsorship from leaders in the field may have his or her work ignored. In still other cases, someone who has learned an important lesson may not consider sharing the results due to lack of time, being unconcerned about whether others gain benefits, or a failure to appreciate the potential of what has been accomplished. In yet other cases, an unconventional, but appropriate, approach may be rejected at first.

Because of such limitations, almost anyone will find that having avid, talented students who stay in touch with their latest findings is another helpful way to stay on top of the latest information and knowledge. If nothing else, such students will often share contacts they have made with individuals and written works that have impressed them as being valuable. Receiving such references will certainly increase the useful breadth of what you can track.

Let us return now to Lesson Fourteen's example of developing and using better measurements and analyses to select more effective baseball players for major-league teams. This time we'll look at the example from the point of view of teaching others and gaining updates as a result.

While it would make a great story to be able to say that such thinking and efforts in baseball had always been directed at better player selection, such is not the case. The original interest in baseball measurements and analysis was based more broadly in seeking to win more games with the players a team already had. For instance, by using statistics to see how each relief pitcher in the team's bullpen typically performed against right-handed batters, a manager could potentially make better decisions about which pitcher to bring in to face a dangerous right-handed batter in a close game. If there were also statistics about how each pitcher had fared against this specific batter, so much the better.

Having been encouraged by the results of using such information, some clubs also began to consider what else could be done. For instance, some teams also used statistics to identify the relative importance of various positions. The result in many cases was to invest more time, money, and effort into having certain kinds of starting pitchers. In the process of working with such pitchers, some of these organizations developed knowledge about how to do so that other teams did not have. For instance, throwing knuckleballs had to be learned from someone who was in his prime in launching the unpredictable pitch. If you had such a person on staff, other pitchers might decide to learn that pitch.

You can see an expression of such a different experiential heritage in how often certain clubs have attracted or developed outstanding starting pitchers with certain qualities. For instance, perhaps vivid memories of Sandy Koufax's left-handed dominance contributed to the Los Angeles Dodgers taking the steps necessary for drafting and developing their amazing lefty Clayton Kershaw. Certainly, it's noteworthy that the Dodgers selected two of their former left-handed pitchers to later be pitching coaches, Ron Perranoski from 1981 to 1994 and Rick Honeycutt from 2006 through the time of this writing. Perranoski pitched for the Dodgers during Koufax's greatest years. Notice, too, that Perranoski was Honeycutt's pitching coach while the latter was on the Dodgers' pitching staff. Could it be that there's some left-handed information and knowledge being passed on here that might not be understood elsewhere? Of course, having Koufax show up at the Dodgers' spring training every year after he retired probably helped reinforce how valuable such knowledge and information can be. Perhaps the once-dominant lefty also passed along his own unique knowledge to several other left-handed pitchers over those years.

New thoughts can come from unexpected directions: As the prior lesson mentioned, fans who understood statistics began to provide their own perspectives of what measurements could help. While the baseball world was at first unimpressed (as were some of the more savvy fans), publication of some fans' new information sparked other fans to add new measurements that extended the initial work in more valuable ways. While one such fan might not deliberately seek to train anyone else, the publications and claims of the initial innovators led to some of such learning.

Improvements made possible by direct teacher-student relationships developed in new ways when baseball clubs began hiring fans who had developed such measurements and new analytical methods to provide input to various kinds of decisions, including player selection. These former-fan teachers then learned from seeing what their baseball students did with the information in operating the actual clubs, and the students learned from the teachers' statistical analyses of the results of the decisions that the consultants had recommended. The former-fan teachers sometimes proposed what seemed to be outlandish ideas, some of which were actually implemented, providing still more opportunities to learn. An example came when consultant Bill James proposed that the Boston Red Sox move away from having a single designated closer, something that the club experimented with in 2003.

James also facilitated more interactions with learners concerning how to use measurements through his online site, Bill James Online (www.billjamesonline.com), a subscriber service that encouraged interactions with him in a question-and-answer format.

While all this teaching and learning would seem like enough to keep any baseball club more than busy gaining useful insights, there was a parallel development that such organizations should also have evaluated: applying new statistics and analyses to player selection and retention for National Football League teams, especially as practiced by Bill Belichick of the New England Patriots. While many professional football teams focused on optimizing performance in each specific position, Belichick sought to optimize the whole team's performance ... especially in light of the potential for injuries and the NFL's salary cap. As an aspect of doing so, he favored identifying and adding players who could contribute through playing more than one position. For instance, a top defensive back might also be part of the punt-coverage squad. An unusually versatile linebacker, Mike Vrabel, occasionally played tight end for the Patriots in red-

Lesson Fifteen: Teach Others and Stay Up-to-Date — An Example

zone situations near the goal line, ultimately catching ten touchdown passes in this role. When the Patriots' defensive secondary was depleted during 2004, a wide receiver near the end of his career, Troy Brown, was converted to play defensive back and provided effectively tight defensive coverage on the opponents' wide receivers, making three interceptions that season.

We can also see evidence of the value of teaching by looking at the NFL executives and coaches who once worked for Belichick. These individuals have often sent valuable recruiting and trade information to their former mentor at the Patriots. Watching some of their teams compete with mutual opponents in Patriot-like ways also provided ideas for game plans that worked well for Belichick's team.

While it would be ideal to select all of your students based on their potential to help you learn while you taught them and then to receive new insights from them for the rest of their lives, for most of us the choices of students to select are limited. You may just have to teach those who show up, trusting that God has sent them for a reason. While you may not always know what God's reasons are, you will be happily surprised from time to time by the learners He has provided.

In my case, I have been blessed to teach many young people in dozens of countries who are unusually passionate about doing the optimal thing, apply enormous energy, and display great curiosity. Teaching them has blessed me by bringing me back to my roots as a young man when I displayed those traits in greater abundance than I am able to do now. In addition, these students reach out to discover things I would never find and provide me with powerful insights that I can apply myself, as well as share with still other students. While I could certainly extend this lesson into being almost half the length of the book, let me remind you that I've reserved all of Part Three for being an effective teacher of breakthrough learning.

So I will stop for now, but just momentarily, as I begin next to more broadly discuss teaching others in Part Three's introduction.

Your Assignments

1. How can teaching others enable you to accomplish more to increase and improve God's Kingdom?

2. What forms of renewal can you gain from your students?

3. What lessons can you learn from keeping in touch with their interests and experiences?

4. What related learning and teaching fields offer insights applicable to your calling from God?

5. What other opportunities does teaching provide you to accomplish more through your own efforts?

Part Three:

Teach Others

My brethren, let not many of you become teachers, knowing that we shall receive a stricter judgment.

For we all stumble in many things. If anyone does not stumble in word, he is a perfect man, able also to bridle the whole body.

Indeed, we put bits in horses' mouths that they may obey us, and we turn their whole body.

Look also at ships: although they are so large and are driven by fierce winds, they are turned by a very small rudder wherever the pilot desires.

Even so the tongue is a little member and boasts great things. See how great a forest a little fire kindles! And the tongue is a fire, a world of iniquity. The tongue is so set among our members that it defiles the whole body,

> *and sets on fire the course of nature; and
> it is set on fire by hell.*
>
> *For every kind of beast and bird,
> of reptile and creature of the sea,
> is tamed and has been tamed by mankind.*
>
> *But no man can tame the tongue.
> It is an unruly evil, full of deadly poison.
> With it we bless our God and Father, and
> with it we curse men,
> who have been made in the similitude of God.
> Out of the same mouth proceed blessing and cursing.*
>
> *My brethren, these things ought not to be so.*
>
> — James 3:1-10 (NKJV)

James 3:1-10 (NKJV) provides worthy cautions about the challenges of teaching. We should always remember that teachers will be judged more strictly by God. In addition, my experience has been that students also judge their teachers more strictly than they do most other people. That's because learners have the reasonable expectation that teachers' behavior, as well as their knowledge and wisdom, will be informative. Teachers are also expected to lecture to students, as well as to answer questions. In doing such speaking, teachers can easily exaggerate something about themselves or their knowledge, as a cheap way to puff up their foolish pride. As such a false sense of superiority grows, teachers can then start to look down on others ... judging, rather than just loving, as Jesus directs us to always do. When such judging begins, disparaging comments may soon follow. And on and on it goes as a "teacher" moves away from the Godly path that Jesus so perfectly modeled.

Such foolishness is usually quite obvious, except perhaps to the person indulging in it. If you doubt that observation, remember the teachers you've had and what things they did that caused you to lose respect for them. I'm sure you won't include in your examples anyone who usually showed you love, kindness, and thoughtful support. However, you'll be quick to remember as bad examples those who usually acted hypocritically, refused to admit errors, or built themselves up at the expense of others. Do you think that any of those people who you remember as bad examples realized how others perceived their behavior? Keep such good and bad examples in mind as you explore the lessons in Part Three, where we divide the steps involved in teaching others into some of the kind of chunks that I've been writing about since Lesson Three.

Lest you feel discouraged by the need to control your tongue in order to avoid the kinds of severe problems James so well describes, let me offer a possible partial antidote: Base any teaching you do on your own carefully developed writing, writing that you exclusively draw on while speaking. I always notice the benefits of taking this approach when teaching. While doing so, I find it easy to stick pretty closely to what I've written in books. That's probably because the Holy Spirit deeply imprinted such messages into my spirit before I ever typed them. In addition, I do a lot of rewriting while preparing the books. I go over every word dozens of times, seeking to improve the writing. Doing so creates a lot of familiarity. In addition, I do most of my own proofreading of the printed text during the production process. To do so, I go slowly over every word in a book once again for a dozen or more additional times. Even with my feeble memory, something is bound to stick after all that rewriting and reviewing. Consequently, I don't make many mistakes while teaching those written subjects, and my tongue doesn't run away from the texts very often.

In addition, I plan and practice understating whatever stories I will tell so that anyone who researches them will find that they are credibly described. While introducing the stories, I make it a habit to apologize in advance for any mistakes I make while speaking. I encourage listeners to challenge what I say, realizing that it's easy for me to be thinking one thing ... and to say the exact opposite. I mentally focus on listeners not as being my students or learners, but rather as being highly capable editors who are helping me to reduce my inevitable errors. If someone challenges me about some aspect of my teaching, I try to take a thankful attitude towards whatever is said ... knowing that at least 10 other people are probably thinking the same thing as what someone just observed. I appreciate that the challenge I just heard can help me to avoid making a bigger fool out of myself than I have already accomplished. Please notice that I take such an approach even when the challenger is totally wrong. After all, I feel grateful because I've just been given a chance to iron out a misunderstanding!

Finally, I begin and end with giving God credit for whatever I say that's correct and taking full blame and responsibility for whatever I say that's incorrect, useless, or otherwise undesirable for any reason. While doing so might seem to encourage me to be careless, I find that this practice focuses me, instead, on representing God as accurately as I can.

Despite all these efforts to avoid mistakes, I'm likely to need to confess sins in this regard to God after teaching, to repent those sins, and to ask Him to strengthen me so that I can do better next time.

Now, if all that sounds okay to you, let me caution you that I do a great deal worse in watching what I say when I'm not teaching something that I have already written in a book. Because I'm aware of this difficulty, I normally caution listeners to such teaching to totally ignore and forget anything I say that doesn't make sense, is wrong, or can't be easily applied. I ask them to only remember and apply what's useful. Notice that I'm putting myself completely in the hands of the hearers' good judgment. Even when I say something sound, I don't expect them to apply it unless the information is useful on its own merits from their perspectives. In teaching, the relationship is not me versus the learner; rather, it's me versus my poor ability to convey what might help someone else, and I desperately need the hearer's help to do so.

If you are confused by the prior paragraph, perhaps it will help you to remember a time when you were unexpectedly asked to give long, complicated directions for someone going somewhere. If you are like me, chances are the unscripted response went something like this: "You go down about a half mile ... you'll pass a Wendy's on the way. Uhhh. Then look for a tall flag pole. Uhhh. When you see it, you're getting closer. After that, there's a hardware store on the far corner. Pass that. Uhhh. Pretty soon you'll get to a pink poodle shop. It's a dress store. Uhhh. I think it's on the left. No, it's on the right. Oh, I'm sorry. It's not on that street at all. Uhhh. Then when you get to Greyson Avenue, start looking for Belle Street on the right. It's just a few blocks up. But remember that the street sign is blocked by a service station sign, so just plan to turn left at the fourth Mobil station you reach. Uhhh. I think it's about 19 blocks and 13 signals from here. ... Have you got that?" Of course, the person will never arrive at this destination unless she or he stops several more times along the way to ask for and receive better directions.

So, when I'm teaching someone else's material, I find that I need to develop a script, keep it with me, and stay focused on it ... to avoid the temptation to ad lib. Now, I like to ad lib, so it's not easy for me to stop doing so. However, I am likely to misstate anything that I haven't carefully scripted. While my talks are much duller as a result of following my scripts, they better teach others useful information.

Let me now give you a more complete description of the lessons in this third part than is found in the book's Introduction. Lesson Sixteen explains how to assist students in developing their learning goals. If you found developing your learning goals during Part One to be at all difficult, you'll benefit by having more empathy while assisting any students who also find this task to be difficult. Hopefully, your own experiences will also help you appreciate and deal with the kinds of stalled thinking that making such goal setting more difficult and time consuming than is necessary.

Lesson Seventeen focuses on explaining a discipline's approach to students, as well as how to apply it. By supplying such an explanation, you'll make learning much easier for your students than you probably experienced while you were developing such knowledge on your own. However, be sure that you also show students how to do such self-learning should they later decide to tackle a different discipline and its applications.

Next, in Lesson Eighteen, you will discover effective tests for identifying what necessary skills, if any, learners lack. Obviously, such tests need to reflect the discipline you are teaching. Again, be sure to prepare students to self-test when they are self-learning other disciplines.

From there, Lesson Nineteen discusses how to demonstrate multiple ways to learn any needed skills. By doing so, you'll enable students to gain such skills faster and obtain more benefits from applying their new knowledge.

Lesson Twenty explains ways of directing learners to practice applying new skills so that their enhanced capabilities will become more permanent. Practicing appropriate chunks of new skills is an important element of doing so. We'll look at ways to identify the best such chunks for a given learner.

In Lesson Twenty-One, we evaluate how to improve the skill-development method for future learners. You'll engage the assistance of your learners to help you make such improvements.

Lesson Twenty-Two shows ways to demonstrate applying the discipline to the learner's goals. Given your knowledge of and experience with the discipline, such a demonstration should be one of the easier and more effective tasks you will do while teaching.

In Lesson Twenty-Three, we describe how to observe and correct any errors in the learner's applications of the discipline to his or her goals. Naturally, the exact ways of doing so will depend on the nature of the learner's difficulties.

From there, Lesson Twenty-Four provides valuable insights into measuring, identifying, and addressing any underlying causes of errors and slowness. Done properly, you will be astonished by how many insights you can develop.

In Lesson Twenty-Five, we explain how to direct a learner to self-improve the process that she or he has been applying. This is one of my favorite activities because I learn so much by doing so, both about the effectiveness of my teaching as well as about how the student perceives what has just been conveyed.

Lesson Twenty-Six demonstrates how learners should be taught to update their awareness of new information and knowledge. Although we have discussed how to do this in several prior lessons, you'll find that helping others to do so is a quite different dimension of this topic.

Finally, in Lesson Twenty-Seven, you are directed to repeat and improve upon the steps you just applied when teaching learners in the future. Naturally, you should rely on the contents of this book. However, you'll want to edit those lessons to better reflect the discipline you've been focusing on, as well as what disciplines a student is likely to learn on her or his own in the future.

Let us now turn to the topic of Lesson Sixteen: Assist Learners to Develop Their Goals.

Lesson Sixteen:

Assist Learners to Develop Their Goals

*May He grant you according to your heart's desire,
And fulfill all your purpose.*

— Psalm 20:4 (NKJV)

Psalm 20:4 (NKJV) reminds us that God has intended a specific purpose for each of us, one that was established before the beginning of the world. In doing so, He also put in our hearts the desire to fulfill each such purpose.

Despite God's good provision in these marvelous ways, many believers cannot easily grasp how to express what and how learning should contribute to enabling them to fulfill their Godly purposes and desires. Such a lack of definition needs to be resolved because others will not be able help these individuals as much as is desirable until after any essential learning goals are clear.

Sometimes the goal-setting difficulties relate to a student not yet knowing what his or her calling is from God. Such an occurrence is especially likely for those who are not yet believers in Jesus. Be patient should that be the case. Perhaps then you will be able use this lesson as a springboard to help someone develop faith in and a relationship with Him.

Lesson Sixteen: Assist Learners to Develop Their Goals

Be open-minded when helping with any such goal setting. After all, you already know certain disciplines. Your presumption, then, might be that you will be helping someone learn one of those disciplines. Not so fast! Depending on what the learner's Godly calling is, you might also need to either learn a new discipline or to refer a learner to someone else who already has good knowledge of and skill in applying such a different discipline. However, rather than assume that you should *always* refer students to someone else for learning a discipline you don't know, remain open to discovering that God might be using a student to encourage you to learn something new, as well.

Before proceeding further in this lesson, I encourage you to re-read Lesson Nine, where you learned how to set goals for applying your new learning. I hope this review will help you better appreciate your learner's perspectives on goal setting.

However, realize that you might also find your teaching can be improved by asking the learner to read this book before receiving your assistance. I make this suggestion mostly because of the potential benefits of having a shared mental framework for the tasks involved, especially by establishing a common vocabulary for discussions. Rather than simply expecting the learner do so on her or his own, you might arrange to have brief conversations during the reading to discuss the material, as well as to answer any questions about what needs to be done or how to accomplish it.

As with Lesson Nine, I encourage your student to begin goal setting by determining what kind of benefits he or she would like to create or increase. Focusing on who should receive benefits is often a fruitful initial step. Such individuals or groups often have problems that need solving or would be helped by having more of some resource. Of course, it's perfectly all right if there is more than one kind of benefit that a learner wants to create or increase. In helping with this part of the thinking, be sure to keep the student focused on narrowing her or his attention to just the aspects of changing someone's situation that will be most beneficial. By looking to add too many different kinds of benefits, the goal-setting task can permanently bog down, never to be completed. If more benefits should be added to the goals after this lesson's work is completed, there will be later opportunities for doing so.

It's not unusual for students who are setting goals to mistakenly project their own circumstances and experiences onto others. A potential way to avoid that error is by having students meet and have discussions about their circumstances and needs with a substantial number of people who will be affected (those I call stakeholders) by the kinds of changes that a student is thinking of accomplishing.

Here's an example. If a student wanted more people to have fluency in at least two languages, it would be easy to focus such a concern around increasing knowledge of two common languages. For example, in the United States, the most commonly spoken languages are English and Spanish. Someone who is a native speaker of one or the other might easily begin focusing on universal fluency for the two. While that might be a worthy goal from the student's perspective, such a goal might seem totally inappropriate to someone who doesn't know either language and has little interest in learning both. Such an individual could be someone who speaks a local language from a small country as well as another global language, say, Portuguese. In this example, the individual is already fluent in two languages. Why should he or she be directed to learn two more? Spending time with those whose language skills differ from knowing either English or Spanish would soon reveal such an issue. If as a result of gaining such understanding the student feels called by God to help more speakers of English or Spanish to learn the other language, the goal could be easily so redefined. However, if the student was serious about making everyone at least fluent in at least one common language in a country, then a different learning goal should be set.

As always, encourage students to pray for guidance from the Holy Spirit while developing their goals, as well as to conduct any research required to understand the likely implications of developing, providing, or increasing the benefits. In considering the language example, I'm sure you appreciate that there are many implications for a society and nation that transcend an individual's needs, implications that could easily sway the choice of benefits to be provided, such as could be accomplished by increasing knowledge of a single common language.

After "who" and "what" have been established in terms of beneficiaries and benefits, encourage your students to carefully consider the timing of "when" the benefits will be provided. Again, the Holy Spirit can be a great resource for doing so. In timing, be sure that your students are realistic in terms of what can be accomplished. For example, in establishing a new solution, quite a bit of effort might have to precede making the attempt, simply in terms of becoming organized. Then, demonstrating the superiority of the solution might have to go on for some longer time before it would become widely understood and accepted. Even after being persuaded by a demonstration, delays will occur in implementation among those who are busy, not very interested, and find it hard to make changes. Considering the timing involved in the past for implementing similar solutions can also provide useful information for setting the timing of accomplishing goals.

As more dimensions of benefits are defined, you can then begin to assist your students to consider what might have to be learned to develop, provide, or increase such benefits. As the scope of learning becomes clearer, those challenges may also influence the students to shift the benefits that are sought to ones that are easier to accomplish. Otherwise, a desire to provide unlimited benefits of all sorts could easily overwhelm the learning capacity of any individual ... except, of course, through the supernatural intervention of the Holy Spirit as instructor.

I hope that you also have a story that reflects your past learning goals to inform your students about how stories can inform and empower their goals. As encouragement, let me share a story I heard just last night that could be connected to a goal of more people becoming dually fluent.

An educator grew up in a family that had lived in the same home since that part of the United States had been part of Mexico. Until the educator's parents' generation, family members had only spoken Spanish. However, a local school had then insisted on teaching her mother only in English. Because they still spoke Spanish at home, the grandparents weren't sure what to do. Because of repeated beatings administered at school to the educator's mother because she spoke in Spanish, the grandparents told their children that they should only speak English. Eventually, the mother's generation lost the ability to speak in Spanish. Since the grandparents knew little English, the communications between the educator's mother and her grandparents had been minimal for many years.

Fortunately, this educator happened to attend a school (the same one her mother had so painfully attended) that then provided the opportunity to learn Spanish through intensive daily immersion. As a result, the educator became the only one in her generation of 117 grandchildren who could speak to the grandparents, something that brought great joy to the grandparents as well as to this granddaughter. Based on that experience, the granddaughter focused her career on making it possible for other youngsters to become dually fluent in English and another language, helping to sustain family connections while also opening the doors to greater career opportunities for the youngsters. As you can imagine, anyone who hears the educator's story immediately appreciates the value of more students having the opportunity to master a second language, whether that language is English or some other one.

While your student may know such a powerful story, he or she may need assistance to make it more compelling to hearers. By helping your student in this way, goal setting and the work to follow will be much more effective. As you help, keep in mind that properly developing the story may also lead your students to improve their learning goals.

Finally, be sure to share with your students any key lessons you gained while setting your learning goals. If, in addition, you've al-

Lesson Sixteen: Assist Learners to Develop Their Goals

ready worked with other students to do such goal setting, draw on those experiences to share other key lessons without compromising the privacy of the prior students.

Your Assignments

1. What does a student need to accomplish to become highly fruitful for increasing and improving God's Kingdom in terms of her or his calling from God?

2. What goals can accurately capture what needs to be done, for whom, and when?

3. Are those goals understandable and encouraging to stakeholders?

4. Do those goals inspire stakeholders to take helpful actions?

5. What stories can improve understanding of the goals and inspire stakeholders to support them?

6. What will the student need to learn for such goals to be accomplished?

Lesson Seventeen:

Explain the Discipline's Approach and How to Apply It

Then Pharaoh said to Joseph:
"Behold, in my dream I stood on the bank of the river.
Suddenly seven cows came up out of the river,
fine looking and fat; and they fed in the meadow.
Then behold, seven other cows came up after them,
poor and very ugly and gaunt,
such ugliness as I have never seen
in all the land of Egypt.

And the gaunt and ugly cows ate up
the first seven, the fat cows.
When they had eaten them up,
no one would have known
that they had eaten them,
for they were just as ugly as at the beginning.

So I awoke. Also I saw in my dream,
and suddenly seven heads came up
on one stalk, full and good.
Then behold, seven heads, withered, thin, and

Lesson Seventeen: Explain the Discipline's Approach and How to Apply It

>
> *blighted by the east wind, sprang up after them.*
> *And the thin heads devoured*
> *the seven good heads.*
>
> *So I told this to the magicians,*
> *but there was no one who could explain it to me."*
>
> *Then Joseph said to Pharaoh,*
> *"The dreams of Pharaoh are one;*
> *God has shown Pharaoh what He is about to do:*
> *The seven good cows are seven years, and*
> *the seven good heads are seven years;*
> *the dreams are one.*
>
> *And the seven thin and ugly cows*
> *which came up after them are seven years,*
> *and the seven empty heads*
> *blighted by the east wind*
> *are seven years of famine.*
>
> *This is the thing which I have spoken to Pharaoh.*
> *God has shown Pharaoh what He is about to do.*
> *Indeed seven years of great plenty will come*
> *throughout all the land of Egypt;*
> *but after them seven years of famine will arise,*
> *and all the plenty will be forgotten*
> *in the land of Egypt;*
> *and the famine will deplete the land.*
> *So the plenty will not be known in the land*
> *because of the famine following,*
> *for it will be very severe.*
> *And the dream was repeated to Pharaoh twice*
> *because the thing is established by God,*
> *and God will shortly bring it to pass.*

> *Now therefore, let Pharaoh select*
> *a discerning and wise man,*
> *and set him over the land of Egypt.*

— Genesis 41:17-33 (NKJV)

To me, Genesis 41:17-33 (NKJV) beautifully demonstrates the kind of gap that can exist between someone who knows a discipline's approach and someone who doesn't. If I had experienced Pharaoh's dream without any explanation, I would probably have simply assumed that it was a nightmare, one I didn't need to take seriously. So it would have taken intervention by the Holy Spirit before I would have sought counsel. Perhaps Pharaoh experienced such a supernatural influence.

Joseph clearly experienced no such difficulties in understanding. Of course, his understanding may have benefited from supernatural influence. Nonetheless, I must admit that his interpretation of the dream seems logical and relevant to me ... even before I consider that the later results closely tracked what he told Pharaoh.

As background for this lesson, I strongly suggest that you reread lessons one and seven. They will remind you of what your learners will need to know about any disciplines that they will be applying.

In thinking about how to teach a discipline to someone else, I must admit to being more strongly influenced by the ways I was introduced to historical approaches than by the instructional techniques used to demonstrate legal and business approaches to me. The contrast was startling to me, due in part to how much more highly regarded the legal and business techniques then were. For instance, when I studied law and business, the two schools were considered to be the foremost pioneers in using case studies to provide practical perspectives and experience in how to perform legal and business analyses. By contrast, the undergraduate history training I received had no particular renown at the time, and I knew little about such training until I was required to undergo it. However, please be aware

Lesson Seventeen: Explain the Discipline's Approach and How to Apply It

that the history department did have a deservedly high reputation for the eminence of its faculty members, their contributions to developing historical methods, and the proliferation of its graduates who were then serving as professors at other universities.

What made the history techniques so much more valuable was that case studies involving primary documents were powerfully supplemented by critical essays by those in the field, as well as by discussions of our reactions to the documents and the essays. I don't recall being exposed to either sort of methodological investigation for applying the recommended approaches to either law or business. In the process of this exposure to historical methods, I came to appreciate some pretty important lessons, ones that are still deeply embedded in my understanding more than a half-century later. For instance, I came to appreciate that although historians attempt to be objective, they are so enmeshed in the perspectives of their time and its ways of thinking that they are actually quite subjective in their approaches.

Having come to believe so, I fully expected that law and business would make the same limiting comments about their disciplines' approaches. While there were occasional hints that some judges and business leaders were being subjective (such as in describing the Supreme Court's difficulties with defining pornography more precisely than "I know it when I see it" and CEOs who came to the top due to being good in selling having a hard time understanding the other functions in a company), both fields seem to treat their approaches as though these were quite close to being objective. In my own view, I didn't see much evidence of there being nearly as much room for objectivity in either law or business as there was in the admittedly subjective work of historians who were trying to be objective.

While I cannot hope to caution you against all the ways that teaching a discipline's approach can be misleading, let me share some of the typical ones. I also hope you'll send me your thoughts to donmitchell@fastforward400.com to help me add perspectives that I should be teaching to others.

First, it's important to appreciate *the limitations of the data* that are being used to apply a discipline's approach. Without doing so, you can end up being deflected from the truth by any arbitrary selectivity that has been applied, without having any clear idea that there's a problem. Historians usually start with what are described as primary documents, ones from the period under study that capture aspects of what was going on then. Such documents can include letters, verbatim texts of interviews with observers, contemporary observations of occurrences, government statistics and records, and any graphic representations drawn from life. Law and business case studies have usually treated their source materials (appellate court decisions and business-school cases) as perfect and complete for the purpose of applying a discipline. However, historians realize that someone simply being there isn't enough to establish truth; you also have to consider the perspective of the source. For instance, even a photograph of an event might be misleading if it was taken from an unhelpful angle or at a time when the evidence was not visible that would have captured what had taken place. While a law or business professor occasionally mentioned a judge's or an executive's limited perspective, those references were few and quite meager. No explanation was ever given of what to do to adjust for a limited perspective. In business-school cases, in particular, there's an editing function involving professors and their assistants writing the cases that creates the equivalent of a subjective layer of gauze over the facts that blurs the reality of what the businesspeople actually were addressing. I have yet to hear anyone in business education say a word about how to handle that latter form of subjectivity.

Second, *what was* no one *looking for?* I find this question to be especially powerful for evaluating scientific investigations. In the interests of being appropriately focused, many scientists narrow their vision of what question to answer to such an extent that they neglect to measure and observe what is actually going on. The problem is somewhat similar to dealing with data limitations, given that not examining in certain ways causes such limitations. For instance, I just read a study of the effects of antibiotics on the immune systems of babies. While I am sure there have been large numbers of studies about babies who take antibiotics, I suspect that few of them considered the long-term effects on the genes that influence immunity, as well as the environment for so-called good bacteria that helps promote health through the digestive system. From reading this new study, I learned that avoiding antibiotics before age 3 can have great lifetime benefits. While all such medications have undergone prior trials to determine whether they are toxic to patients or cause harmful side effects, no government requires testing for other kinds of potentially harmful effects. In part, realize that such limitations occur because of how ignorant we might be about a given area of science. For example, knowledge about what some genes do in humans has only recently been developed.

Third, *what are the biases inherent in the data that no one is going to warn you about?* A good example can be found in the cultural forms of ignorance present at a point in time. For instance, although scientists have known a great deal about heredity since Gregor Mendel did his work, until DNA was thoroughly studied many aspects of how heredity actually works were ignored ... such as the ability of some genes to turn themselves on or off based on the environment that is encountered. So if you look at work about heredity until quite recently, you'll find potential lessons obscured by such ignorance that affected how the research questions were posed.

Fourth, *what are the best questions to ask?* Let me share with you here one of my favorite examples. If you ask the question of how poverty originated for an individual, you may not gain very much useful information about how poverty could be eliminated for that same person. Think about the differences between asking about the causes and identifying solutions in another context. For instance, if you grew out of shape due to spending too much time studying in college, simply stopping such studies won't get you back into shape. A different solution is needed.

Fifth, *where can you obtain the best information?* Many people skip thinking about this subject. Instead, they just look around for where it's easiest to do so. To me, that's like only looking for a lost key at night in places where there happen to be street lights.

While I could offer other insights, it's better if you come up with your own, ones that reflect your understanding of and experience with a discipline and its approaches. After that, find ways to introduce your students to working with the primary data that can best inform an accurate and effective analysis. Here's where I had some bones to pick with my history professors and instructors: They only seemed to provide data that were too limited to be of much value. Whenever I asked how to round out what I had read, they would sheepishly admit that they were aware of other sources that enabled them to draw certain conclusions but didn't want me to use those sources. How was I to do a proper job without seeing those sources? Well, I couldn't. I suspect that this faulty preparation of materials turned me against wanting to become a historian. I ran into a similar problem while doing my own historical research with primary materials as an undergraduate. Despite having tutors for two years who had deep experiences with primary sources in my field, neither of them explained to me what other primary sources could have been helpful and how to access those materials. I did the best I could with newspaper reports, but it was obvious that they were a poor source of insights.

Because of such difficulties, unless there is a necessary reason to look at older sources, in many cases for the purpose of explaining the discipline you would do better to work with a student to develop new information by using the best data-development methods. In many scientific fields, however, doing so may not be practical. If specialized, essential equipment is not available, for instance, perhaps you could arrange to simulate some data in a way that will closely resemble having actual material, while avoiding the need to go to great expense and effort for doing so.

Lesson Seventeen: Explain the Discipline's Approach and How to Apply It

Before applying either high quality real or simulated data, I also encourage you to slowly and deliberately talk your student through a full example of employing the discipline. Ideally, such an example should be based on some work you've done. Because of your familiarity with the example, you'll be able to add details and answer questions that your student will find to be valuable. However, feel free to abbreviate the example so that you don't repeat steps that are essentially identical. In this way, you might be able to encapsulate what took many weeks into a thorough description of the elements of each step during only a few hours. As you do, keep an open mind about how long the description should take. Your student may want you to slow down and go into elaborate details in places where the application is somewhat counterintuitive or confusing. Take whatever time is needed to eliminate any misunderstandings, discomfort, and confusion before proceeding.

Next, give your student some problems that provide the opportunity to use data. Such problems don't need to address every aspect of the application, just the aspects that are critical or likely to cause errors.

After the student becomes familiar with applying good data, then you will be able to introduce flawed data. Then the student can apply the kinds of challenging questions I've posed so far in this lesson in ways that are relevant to the approaches of the discipline being learned. From such experiences, the student can graduate to looking at the pros and cons of alternative methods described in published studies, determining for her- or himself which of these approaches have been more fruitful.

Finally, I suggest that you take the student through the many steps you undoubtedly followed to develop your own knowledge about the discipline's approaches. In doing so, encourage students to repeat any activities you did that were particularly insightful.

Before leaving this lesson, I also urge you to have a general discussion with the student about how this learning process might be repeated for a related discipline's approaches, should the student decide to learn those, as well, through his or her own efforts. If you have the skill to do so, you might also provide some limited problems that a student is likely to encounter in self-learning how to apply a different discipline.

Your Assignments

1. What are the most important lessons that you want your students to learn about the limitations of the discipline's approaches?

2. What are the best ways for a student to experience and develop an appreciation for such limitations?

3. How can students experience and develop an understanding of the strengths of a discipline's approaches?

4. What practical applications does a student need to make before becoming competent in a discipline?

5. How can you give students a strong sense of how to learn a different discipline's approaches on their own?

Lesson Eighteen:

Test Learners for Necessary Skills

*Now it came to pass after these things that
God tested Abraham, and said to him, "Abraham!"*

And he said, "Here I am."

*Then He said, "Take now your son, your only son Isaac,
whom you love, and go to the land of Moriah, and
offer him there as a burnt offering
on one of the mountains of which I shall tell you."*

*So Abraham rose early in the morning
and saddled his donkey, and
took two of his young men with him, and Isaac his son;
and he split the wood for the burnt offering, and
arose and went to the place of which God had told him.*

*Then on the third day Abraham lifted his eyes
and saw the place afar off.
And Abraham said to his young men,
"Stay here with the donkey; the lad and I will go yonder
and worship, and we will come back to you."*

Lesson Eighteen: Test Learners for Necessary Skills

*So Abraham took the wood of the burnt offering and
laid it on Isaac his son; and
he took the fire in his hand, and a knife, and
the two of them went together.*

*But Isaac spoke to Abraham his father and said,
"My father!"*

And he said, "Here I am, my son."

*Then he said, "Look, the fire and the wood, but
where is the lamb for a burnt offering?"*

*And Abraham said, "My son, God will provide
for Himself the lamb for a burnt offering."*

So the two of them went together.

*Then they came to the place
of which God had told him.
And Abraham built an altar there and
placed the wood in order; and he bound Isaac
his son and laid him on the altar, upon the wood.
And Abraham stretched out his hand
and took the knife to slay his son.*

But the Angel of the LORD *called to him
from heaven and said, "Abraham, Abraham!"*

So he said, "Here I am."

*And He said, "Do not lay your hand on the lad,
or do anything to him;
for now I know that you fear God,
since you have not withheld your son,
your only son, from Me."*

Then Abraham lifted his eyes and looked, and
there behind him was
a ram caught in a thicket by its horns.
So Abraham went and took the ram, and
offered it up for a burnt offering instead of his son.

And Abraham called the name of the place,
The-LORD-Will-Provide; as it is said to *this day,*
"In the Mount of the LORD it shall be provided."

— Genesis 22:1-14 (NKJV)

Fortunately, your students probably won't have to undergo any tests nearly as demanding as the one that God used to determine Abraham's faithfulness. However, please realize that skill tests are essential for ensuring that your students can effectively apply a discipline.

I was recently reminded of the importance of such tests when a student approached me about how to improve his critical reading and writing skills so that he could learn about the forms of philosophy that are related to science, technology, engineering, and math. As you might imagine, no one had previously presented me with such a request. After reviewing my readings in these fields, I quickly appreciated that he was going to be undertaking quite a substantial amount of study. I also recalled how relatively impenetrable some of the writings are. How could I best help him?

Since God had kindly provided me with the assignment to write this lesson at almost the same time, I quickly appreciated that starting with understanding his current skills would help. In the process, I also asked him if he felt comfortable developing his reading and writing skills by working with such philosophy materials. He eagerly agreed.

Since there are many ways to test reading and writing, I decided it would be good to know more about what education he had already completed. He reported that he was a high school graduate.

Lesson Eighteen: Test Learners for Necessary Skills

Since I often assist students with college-entrance examinations and admission applications, I quickly appreciated I could use portions of such tests to gauge his skill levels. By using such tests, I would be able to interpret the results compared to the norm of those who attend various kinds of colleges, for similarities and differences to other students I have taught, and in terms of the kinds of mistakes that he made. I quickly developed such a custom test.

While doing so, I had to make a decision: Should I test for how much math he could understand? That question arose because some writings that interested him required appreciating mathematical expressions, problems, and approaches. Realizing that his overall reading and writing skills might be inadequate to initially comprehend such more difficult materials, I decided against such initial testing for him. Why? He has plenty to learn, and developing his math skills would be accelerated by first helping him become a better reader.

I felt comfortable taking this approach because of realizing that I could quickly overcome any mistake I had made in this regard by giving him a one-hour math test at any time. A benefit of not doing so now was to reduce any discouragement he might feel about his test results. My experience has been that people tend to be more pessimistic about their ability to learn better ways to do math than they are for learning to be better readers or writers.

Because you already understand the discipline that your student wants to apply, as well as which applications will be most relevant to the student's learning goals, you should be in a good position to define a simple set of tests to tell you what skills your student needs to learn. You, too, may be able to use portions of standardized tests to assess current skill and knowledge levels.

In doing such testing, I also encourage you to consider whether the testing can be spaced out over time. For instance, if you are going to be teaching the student for several months, you can make the beginning less difficult by reducing the initial testing. I suggest you consider ways to test that will pick up the minimum, rather than the maximum, information about a student's skills. Doing so will further reduce the need for initial testing. After all, you will be guiding the student to apply a process before you are done teaching, and during such an application you will have many opportunities to pick up on any minor skill deficiencies.

One skill I urge you to test sooner rather than later is how effectively a student seeks help. You can test that ability, in part, by making some of your directions slightly incomplete, as a way to see if he or she will come back with questions. You should also ask the student to find some examples of the discipline being applied, so you can learn about her or his research abilities.

After that, feel free to draw on problems that you've encountered in your own learning and application of the discipline that will demonstrate any lack of skills. As you interpret any results, be sure to keep in mind that your student will be able to engage the assistance of others who are reasonably available to fill in for any personal skill gaps. For instance, if a student writes reasonably well in terms of content but lacks a good grasp of grammar and punctuation, I can simply encourage that student to work with an editor. In the process of doing so, the student would gradually become a better writer, and all of the writing in the meantime would ultimately be improved to adequate quality.

Before finishing the testing, I also encourage you to describe your self-testing activities while you learned the discipline on your own (as described in Part Two). Discuss with your student how such a process might be done by him or her during a separate self-learning activity for a different discipline. If you are good at developing your own self-testing questions, also prepare a few that might be used by your student to test for skills needed for applying a related discipline.

Your Assignments

1. What skills will your student need to develop for applying the discipline that cannot be readily accessed in some other way?

Lesson Eighteen: Test Learners for Necessary Skills

2. What tests can determine how much skill your student has in these necessary areas?

3. How can such tests be made simple and easy?

4. How can you use the test results to determine how much learning and of what sort will be required to fill in for any deficiencies in necessary skills?

Lesson Nineteen:

Demonstrate Multiple Ways to Learn Skills

*But now the righteousness of God
apart from the law
is revealed, being witnessed by
the Law and the Prophets,
even the righteousness of God,
through faith in Jesus Christ,
to all and on all who believe.*

*For there is no difference;
for all have sinned and
fall short of the glory of God,
being justified freely by His grace
through the redemption that is in Christ Jesus,
whom God set forth
as a propitiation by His blood,
through faith,
to demonstrate His righteousness,
because in His forbearance
God had passed over the sins
that were previously committed,*

Lesson Nineteen: Demonstrate Multiple Ways to Learn Skills

> *to demonstrate at the present time*
> *His righteousness,*
> *that He might be just and the justifier*
> *of the one who has faith in Jesus.*
>
> — Romans 3:21-26 (NKJV)

As the Bible so powerfully demonstrates, God loves us and wants to be in a good relationship with us. He first did this by creating Adam and Eve and putting them in a perfect world. When they disobeyed by eating fruit from the tree of the knowledge of good and evil, He didn't destroy them. When their descendants became horribly rebellious and decadent after several generations, God still rescued Noah and his family so He could start again with humans. After Noah's descendants also turned out badly in many cases, God tried once again for a good relationship, this time with Abraham and his descendants, choosing to bless them despite their sins. After rescuing Abraham's descendants from Pharaoh, God provided for them in the desert and brought the descendants of the emancipated ones to the Promised Land. To help them understand what righteousness is, He gave them the Mosaic Law. Once in the Promised Land, the Hebrews again disappointed Him by worshiping other so-called gods. He sent these idolaters into exile in Babylon, yet remained present with them there and later brought back a remnant to the Promised Land. Then, after the descendants of the remnant also became rebellious, God provided His most magnificent demonstration of love by sending His Son to live, die, and be resurrected so that *all* can choose to be in a righteous relationship with God. Despite these amazing demonstrations of God's love, holiness, and faithfulness, many people today prefer to disobey Him, some of them even denying that He exists ... despite all of the historical and present evidence of His existence and goodness.

Similarly, we should expect that much of what we demonstrate to students about learning necessary skills will not initially be understood and acted on. If we take the point of view that we should keep trying, however, then all will be well. If, instead, we act as if only one or two ways to learn are appropriate for others, we can expect most students to have many ongoing, unresolved difficulties in developing their skills.

As a first step to help someone learn, it's hard to beat asking the student to describe all of her or his various successful and unsuccessful learning experiences. The only difficulty you may encounter in doing so is that some people either won't understand or remember very much about what worked and what did not about their past learning. In such cases, I've usually been able to elicit more details by asking some pointed questions. Here are a few questions that might help you to do so:

- Do you like to learn in a classroom with many other people or individually in a quiet place?
- Do you prefer to listen to lectures or to have discussions?
- What kinds of written materials are easiest for you to use?
- Do you prefer to ask questions or to answer them about the material you are learning?
- What makes you feel uncomfortable while learning?
- What can disrupt your learning?
- What kind of learning assignments do you find to be most difficult?
- What is hardest for you to learn? Why?

Many people learn best from having just one narrow type of interaction with information, such as one that just emphasizes seeing things, having a discussion, or physically experiencing what is involved. Many people are aware of their differential abilities in these regards and seek to maximize their most effective learning styles. If your student is not aware of his or her best learning mode, be ready to demonstrate at least these three ways of either learning new skills or building on existing ones. Also be prepared to demonstrate com-

Lesson Nineteen: Demonstrate Multiple Ways to Learn Skills

binations of all three learning interactions. Although someone may initially prefer one narrow type of learning over the other two that are demonstrated, almost everyone will gain even more understanding by receiving additional perspectives through interacting with the other two learning modes. In the process, a learner will probably also increase her or his future ability to benefit from the other two modes for interacting with information and knowledge.

Other useful connections can be added to the learning demonstrations, such as relevance to something that interests the student. For instance, a learner who wants to eliminate poverty will apply much more attention to and gain greater understanding from a learning demonstration that includes actually assisting a poor person to greatly increase income or to substantially decrease living costs. A demonstration that also involves something with which the student is familiar can be even more helpful. Simulations of everyday experiences can dramatically demonstrate to a learner the benefits of developing a skill or not doing something that interferes with properly applying such a skill.

In demonstrating learning methods, always expect the student to misunderstand part of what is shown, said, or experienced. That is only natural. None of us can fully absorb all the relevant information the first time we see, hear, or experience it. Consequently, the learning method a student prefers after seeing a demonstration may not, in fact, be the best one for him or her. To test the relevance of a student's initial preference after learning a few aspects of skills with the indicated method ask the student to then perform a few simple tasks. If all goes well, such a learning method is probably appropriate. Of course, if matters go poorly, you will soon realize the need to substitute some other learning method.

What if at that point the demonstrations have exhausted your repertoire of teaching with different learning methods? Well, there is always another way. Politely ask the student for time to formulate some more learning alternatives. In so doing, you should be humble and expect to be and to feel humbled. Students like their teachers to be all-knowing, but, of course, no human ones are. However, you can eventually develop some fine respect in your student's eyes by being willing to start afresh in a new direction and then succeeding in doing so.

I have experienced my share of needing to locate new ways for someone to learn needed skills. Let me describe what it was like. After first thinking that I had no idea of what to do next, I eventually reconsidered my notes about how a student had responded to each demonstration method. Rarely did I find that nothing worked during a learning demonstration. In fact, almost everything might have gone great, but the net result might still have been a washout. By considering where each method flopped, I can sometimes perceive a way to combine the methods so that only the functional parts of two or more prior demonstrations are retained. When the successful elements of different methods can be combined into one, successful learning almost always follows.

In some instances, I've been pleasantly surprised when a student later reported that she or he now "gets it" after having the benefit of sleeping on and thinking about the prior demonstrations for a few days. Nevertheless, in such instances I'll still demonstrate any promising combination method, and I almost always find that a student will prefer it to a previously demonstrated one that now "works."

What if there is no obvious way to only combine successful elements of various learning methods? Well, such times are made for bringing us teachers closer to God so He can demonstrate more ways that He cares for and looks after us. After seeking His direction in prayer, my mind has always been filled with some novel possibility that connected various things that the student had told me, shown through her or his behavior, or that I was aware of from the context of the student's life. The process of making those connections has often seemed to me as if I were putting together a complex jigsaw puzzle. I would begin to sense elements of connections that fit perfectly together. As I added one piece of a learning process to a piece of another one, I would begin to see a bigger picture. Eventually, the stu-

Lesson Nineteen: Demonstrate Multiple Ways to Learn Skills

dent and I could see, hear, and touch one large, continuous image of a wonderful learning method for that individual.

However, in such cases I have always proceeded very gently and tentatively to present the new way of learning. Let me describe how I did so in an individual case. I first mentioned that I had thought of something that might work, but I also said that I had never tried the method with anyone else. Before any demonstrating, I asked for the student's patient indulgence while I presented my idea and explained why it might work. When the student said to go ahead, I then proceeded to explain and demonstrate one little step at a time. After each step, I asked again if it was all right to go on to the next step. I took my time, perhaps even going a little slower than the student would have preferred. I did so because I didn't want the student to feel rushed or manipulated in any way. I encouraged the student to describe how experiencing the demonstration felt as I continued. I made notes of anything that didn't seem to go smoothly.

Most such demonstrations have been successful. When they have not worked as intended, I've then asked the student if I might make some adjustments for what did not work and then test the revised method at another time. In such circumstances, students have usually shared with me some added details of what they liked and didn't like about the demonstration. With that information in hand, I have always then been able to make further refinements that enabled the student to learn effectively.

You might find that a learning method doesn't work, even after making such refinements. Don't give up. Ask the student if you can try again. Be sure to give yourself enough time to absorb and think about what you've been learning about how to be most helpful to this student before proposing anything else. If you still feel stuck at such a point, feel free to contact me (donmitchell@fastforward400.com) so that we can pray, talk, and think through the choices together.

Your Assignments

1. What learning method does the student prefer?

2. What learning methods does this student want you to avoid?

3. How can more learning methods be added to the preferred one or ones without diluting the student's focus?

4. What problems did you notice the student experiencing while trying the various learning methods?

5. What worked best during each of the method demonstrations?

6. How might aspects of the different demonstrated methods be combined for better learning?

Lesson Twenty:

Drill Learners in Skills and Track Their Progress

*And now, little children, abide in Him,
that when He appears, we may have confidence
and not be ashamed before Him at His coming.
If you know that He is righteous, you know
that everyone who practices righteousness
is born of Him.*

— 1 John 2:28-29 (NKJV)

The New King James Version of the Bible doesn't include the word "drill." With the Holy Spirit's help, I've selected the phrase "practices righteousness" from 1 John 2:29 (NKJV) to indicate the meaning I intend for you to associate with *drill* in this lesson: Repeat doing the right thing for expanding and improving God's Kingdom. Then you will abide in practicing righteousness.

I begin with this explanation because for many people a "drill" has unfortunate connotations. If I mention that word to my wife, she imagines painful time spent in a dentist's chair. If I had mentioned *drill* to my dad, he would have recalled unpleasant, dangerous times while in the U.S. Army. As an elementary-school student, I associated *drill* with an air raid siren going off, triggering an evacua-

Lesson Twenty: Drill Learners in Skills and Track Their Progress

tion to a bomb shelter that protected us very little from a potential nuclear attack.

My alternate word, "practices," often has negative connotations in the Bible, as well. In many instances, verses including *practices* refer to various ways of engaging in extreme wickedness. However, in everyday language the word *practices* does not normally have any such connotation. The word most often comes up in the context of developing skill in sports or performing.

So as you read this lesson, please take out a mental eraser and eliminate any negative connotations that occur in your mind concerning *drill* and *practices*. Thank you!

Okay, you probably realize that I must have a good reason for choosing to use the words *drill* and *practices*. Yes, I do. When I work with students who are learning new subjects, they immediately understand that "to drill" or "to practice" means repeatedly using helpful methods until they become useful habits. So that's a good start. Many people immediately know what I mean when I use the verb form of *drill* in a learning context, rather than the word as a noun. An even better attribute of mentioning the word is that such students almost always smile and look more enthusiastic after I inform them that they will *drill* to become better at performing some task they have just begun to learn. In other words, *to drill* is often viewed positively when connected to learning something a student seeks to master.

If you don't happen to have a positive reaction to being directed *to drill*, I apologize for making you uncomfortable. Feel free to substitute some other word that has positive associations for you. For example, if *to practice* or *practices* has a positive connotation for you, just substitute either choice from now on.

Let me add another thought: Don't just drill, *drill in small, relevant chunks*. That direction is probably unclear to you. Let me explain what I mean in terms of an example related to my work with high-school math students.

Breakthrough Learning

While learning algebra, many students do quite well with solving combinations of simultaneous equations and inequalities where each expression contains two unknowns, ones that are often labeled as "x" and "y." Perhaps that reference brings back memories of substituting the value of one variable (defined in terms of the other variable in one equation) into the second, simultaneous equation (meaning that the two equations have a common solution, a place where their lines cross on a graph). Alternatively, you might be reminded of adding or subtracting with two equations or inequalities to first eliminate one variable, and then plugging the resulting value for the other variable into one of the original equations or inequalities to determine a value for the initially eliminated variable.

However, if a student hasn't applied either solution technique in two or more years, my experience has been that the student is highly likely to have forgotten them both. In such cases, students will just stare at the simultaneous equations (or inequalities) and feel frustrated. Why? Well, most American schools are now so focused on students learning math *concepts* at ever-younger ages that the curricula don't assign nearly enough practice for students to permanently develop skill in *applying* the concepts. Instead, quick understanding is gained that's sufficient to pass a test or a course, and that's the end of working on such problems.

If I next show such a blankly staring student an algebraic expression that involves *f(x)*, a feeling of sheer panic may overwhelm the student's mind. If, however, I then remind her or him that *f(x)* simply means the "y" value that they are used to seeing in an equation or inequality, he or she will immediately relax and smile. Now, you would think that using one way to express an unknown value would be immediately appreciated as being the equivalent of any other way of expressing an unknown value. Not so! Students don't usually understand the reasons why certain ways of expressing mathematical concepts are employed. In the case of *f(x)*, it's a convenient way to focus on how the value of an expression changes as different values for the unknown ("x" in this case) are substituted. Thus, *f(x)* = $x + 5$

Lesson Twenty: Drill Learners in Skills and Track Their Progress

has a value of 6 when *x* has a value of 1 *f(1)* (substituting "1" for "*x*" on the right side of the equation), and the same expression has a value of 10 when *x* has a value of 5 *f(5)* (substituting "5" for "*x*" on the right side of the equation).

I apologize if I've made you uncomfortable by using this example. Hopefully, you remember enough algebra to find the references relevant and meaningful, whether or not you can actually make the calculations I've just referenced.

Please bear with me a little longer as I now detail an example of *how to drill in relevant chunks*. For solving two simultaneous equations containing the same two variables, I might first introduce the idea of the two lines crossing one another as a way to demonstrate a common solution. As a first step in such an introduction, I might request a student to graph the two equations as lines. Some students might have trouble doing so. If so, I would reduce the chunk by asking the student to put one point from one equation on a graph. If she or he had trouble with that, I would reduce the chunk further by suggesting putting on a point where either *x* or *y* was equal to zero, as a way to simplify the calculations. If he or she still could not do that, I would make the chunk still smaller by asking the student to substitute the value of zero for one of the unknowns in the simpler of the two equations and then calculate the remaining value for the other unknown. If more difficulties arose in doing so, I would break down what's needed into smaller steps, such as explaining how to add and subtract from both sides of the equation to simplify the expression. After doing so successfully, a student still might not understand what to do with the resulting *x* and *y* values. If that were the case, I would chunk down into how to turn these two bits of information into a point on a graph. If the student couldn't then draw and correctly label the axes for an *x-y* graph, I would chunk down into teaching the individual acts required for doing so.

I'm sure by now you get the idea: Many tasks require a substantial number of skills or applying several different pieces of information and knowledge, each of which has to be put in the right sequence to obtain the correct result. Dividing tasks into smaller, sequential chunks is a very useful way to find out what parts of the task a learner hasn't yet mastered.

Once having found a useful chunk of a task that a student needs to master, the next step is to have a student drill in performing that chunk. Let me explain what I mean by continuing with this lesson's algebra example.

Let's assume that the relevant drilling chunk for a student is finding a value for one of the unknowns and then substituting that value into the other simultaneous equation. While not knowing how to do so might seem unlikely to you if you are good at math, I promise you that many people who are quite intelligent do not remember how to make such substitutions.

I find that the most effective drilling occurs when a student is in charge of setting up the problems. To demonstrate how to do so, I would ask a student to take a problem that has just been solved and then to make just one change to one of the equations. Such a first change might be to change a constant from "5" to "6." Obviously, that's a trivial change. However, students feel good about trying to solve a problem after making such a change. The student can look back at what was just done to see where the constant fits and then substitute a different constant. Most people will then get the problem right on the first try. If not, I can quickly point out what's been done wrong due to a misunderstanding. I go on to explain the proper method in a different way.

After that, I'll encourage a student to make a bigger change in constants. Doing so might mean changing "5" into "10." Some students initially look uncomfortable, but they are then pleasantly surprised to find that they can do it.

Once comfort and facility are gained with such changes, I'll ask a student to make a large change in constants, say, by changing "5" into "100." This step usually goes well. I'll keep nudging the student until some very large numbers are substituted into one of the equations.

Lesson Twenty: Drill Learners in Skills and Track Their Progress

Now, in some cases, the outcome will be that the two equations aren't simultaneous any more. That can occur when two equations are parallel to one another. I'll warn the student that doing this drilling can occasionally have such an effect. When a student notices that such an event has occurred, the experience becomes a source of delight for her or him, rather than a source of confusion or frustration.

Once constants have been changed in many ways and the calculations done correctly, I'll shift to having changes made to the variables. Thus, "$2x$" might be substituted for "x." And so on, as with scaling up the sizes of changes to the constants.

After that, I'll encourage the student to make changes in the constants and variables in both equations. I love seeing the enthusiasm that students usually bring to such a task. They now feel confident about what once intimidated them!

When skill has been gained in solving problems involving different constants and variables in both equations, I'll challenge the student to create completely new sets of simultaneous equations that look quite different from the ones that were the basis for the initial drilling. Most students will branch out slowly. After a while, the student will graduate to creating equations with much different variables and constants. At this point, students start to have an intuitive sense of what simultaneous equations look like and how they work together.

When such confidence and knowledge are gained, I'll encourage a student to add a third set of variables, but to do so in a way that the problem can still be solved solely for simultaneous, constant values of x and y. One way to do so, for instance, is to have the third variables cancel one another out as you add or subtract the equations, so it's as if the third variables don't exist.

At some point, I'll direct a student to do similar work with inequalities, if equations were the first focus ... or vice versa.

As you can see, it takes a bit of ongoing discussion to help a student appreciate how to drill in ways that create confidence and mastery. You might be wondering if this kind of interaction has to be repeated. In most cases, showing someone how to properly drill in a subject will allow the student to then develop other, relevant drills without assistance. However, you should expect to be asked an occasional question. I rarely receive any of such questions after someone has drilled at least three times following discussions with me. So repetition will eventually enable your student to master the new skill of designing helpful drills!

Your Assignments

1. What steps in a task is a student unable to do?

2. What is the student confused about?

3. How can breaking the task down into smaller chunks help?

4. Once the proper chunks have been identified for developing mastery, how can drilling for those chunks best be done?

5. What would be a good sequence of adding complications for a student to deal with while drilling?

6. How can the student be prepared to repeat such drilling for relevant chunks concerning other tasks?

Lesson Twenty-One:

Adjust the Skill-Learning Method

If the ax is dull,
And one does not sharpen the edge,
Then he must use more strength;
But wisdom brings success.

— Ecclesiastes 10:10 (NKJV)

Many people fail to appreciate when repetition is counterproductive, such as when someone is cutting down trees with a dull ax. Because meeting a critical deadline can sometimes mean taking shortcuts that involve serious drawbacks, we should be careful to avoid doing so when possible. For instance, since the essence of teaching someone breakthrough learning is making him or her vastly more productive, we should avoid giving the impression that necessary maintenance for doing so should be skipped.

I recently heard a story that provides an expensive metaphor for why we need to properly maintain our learning. Two highly educated people shared the use of a vehicle. Each person knew that the other one was well aware that the engine oil needed to be changed from time to time. However, each one assumed that the other one, an equally responsible person, would do so. Neither one did. The vehicle was driven for so many months without an oil change that

Lesson Twenty-One: Adjust the Skill-Learning Method

the oil started turning into sludge. After enough sludge had developed, a sensor light went on indicating that the vehicle was low on oil. Since the light flickered on and off from time to time as the sludge moved around, both responsible people ignored it ... until, that is, the engine seized up and was ruined. Yes, they saved some time and money by not checking and changing the oil, but the new vehicle they purchased to replace the old one cost over $30,000. Don't make that kind of mistake!

Failing to adjust a skill-learning method can be even more expensive than the $30,000 paid for a new vehicle in this example. We are dealing here with something that economists often call "opportunity costs." Let me explain. If I have a dollar, I can keep it or spend it. If I keep it, it has a value of a dollar. If I spend it for a lottery ticket that wins me $500 million, spending the dollar has increased my value by $500 million minus one dollar. In a world where I have perfect information about the future, not buying that lottery ticket (I don't recommend that you actually make such a purchase, since the odds are poor that you'll even get your money back) in my example has an opportunity cost equal to the lost opportunity ($500 million) minus the cost of accessing the opportunity ($1). Got it? If not, send me an e-mail to donmitchell@fastforward400.com, and I'll explain in a different way.

Most people don't feel poorer when they miss opportunities because they never felt that they had the benefit. Consequently, missing an opportunity can feel like missing nothing, rather than taking a large actual loss, one that could be much more expensive than destroying a vehicle's engine.

Okay, now you might be wondering (I know I would be) why a skill-learning method might need adjustment. Let me share an example to explain. In most skill areas, mistakes are most often made in the more fundamental chunks of the tasks. As a result, not knowing how to do a few things could cause almost every result to be wrong. It's not unusual, for instance, for math students to forget how to subtract a negative number (say, -5) from a positive one (say 5). The difference is 10. Many students will come up, instead, with either zero or -10 as an answer. Once this form of subtraction can be done correctly, such errors will disappear.

If a student has difficulty and requires a long time to learn this chunk, the resulting process learned might contain several checking steps. For instance, the student might be checking to see if she or he is subtracting the correct number from the other number, rather than reversing them. (If you subtract 5 from -5, the answer is -10). Then, the student might also be doing the math on a calculator to check any work done by hand. The calculator checking might be repeated to test for errors in punching in the numbers. There might also be a step for checking that negative signs were written down correctly. And so forth.

Notice, however, that many of those checking steps can be eliminated once a student is quite competently subtracting any negative numbers from positive ones. Think of making such adjustments as being somewhat like removing the training wheels from a bicycle as a youngster learns to balance without them. The youngster can then go faster and to more places. Your student may well be able to do something similar.

Adjustments to reduce unnecessary checking aren't the only ones that are likely to be needed. As students gain effectiveness in breakthrough learning, overall competence may grow to the point that they can benefit from applying quite different steps, ones that take full advantage of a newly developed skill. For instance, as a student gains insight into how permutations in the steps for applying a skill affect the results and how much time and effort are required to obtain them, a useful, new step might be added for identifying untested, potentially more effective permutations of the application. From the results of such an analysis, a student might then postulate some permutations to test. From such testing, a whole new set of steps might be added to explore more significant possibilities, even before the student attempts to master performing the most accepted version of the application. In such a case, a student might leapfrog well past

Lesson Twenty-One: Adjust the Skill-Learning Method

the best of what has been done previously without ever needing to learn any of the soon-to-be obsolete methods.

As a different example, a student who is teaching others might develop a new way to test skills that also simultaneously demonstrates the correct ways to perform these skills, combined in just one process. Such a more effective result might be accomplished by having students test their skills on a computer loaded with a program that automatically redirects the learner who makes a mistake to materials that cover the basics for performing that task. Done in an extremely effective way, such a testing-and-teaching method might enable neophytes to be completely competent during the initial time they are tested for a new skill.

Naturally, you will have noticed where a given student had difficulties with the skill-learning method that you used. Such difficulties will always be present in at least some activities, no matter how well a skill-learning method works compared to the alternatives that have been used previously. Be sure to probe the learner for the reasons why such difficulties might be occurring.

My experience has been that some learners have no idea of what created the difficulty. However, they are usually good at describing what they were thinking and experiencing before, during, and after the difficulty occurred.

Consequently, I find it can be highly effective to watch learners while they apply a learning method. As I do, I measure as much as I can about what's going on, limited only to avoiding anything that would make them feel self-conscious or uncomfortable.

Here are some of the things that I might observe and measure:

- How long does each step take?
- How does the duration differ from an efficient rate?
- How does the duration of the step relate to the accuracy of how well it is done?
- What has the learner done during the step?
- How does the learner's body shift during the step?

- How does the learner's expression change?
- When does anxiety seem to occur?
- When is the learner doing activities that aren't likely to help?

As a follow-up to making these observations and measurements, I then show the learner where unusual activities or results occurred. I take note of any associations that could indicate links between possible causes and effects.

While it can be tempting to only chunk down such discussions into specific topics, I find that there are likely to be connections between topics that relate to broader causes that need to be addressed. For instance, someone's having forgotten how to do a key task can affect quite a few of such measurements.

Learners are usually surprised by what the measurements demonstrate. By sharing such measurements, the perspectives of the learner and teacher can move much closer together. The measurements also make it possible to test adjustments by measuring how well a student performs while using an adjusted learning process.

So what kinds of adjustments are likely to be needed? While it would take far more space than this book offers to deal with even a small fraction of the useful possibilities, it may help you if I provide a few examples.

Let me focus on learners who are somewhere near average or slightly above in their ability to apply the learning approach, a skill level that applies to a large percentage of learners. My experience has been that such students will vary a great deal in their mix of abilities. While overall they might be near average, in specific aspects such a student might vary from almost incompetent to being outstanding.

Such variations, when they are present, often call for adjusting skill-learning methods to simplify and slow them where a learner has difficulties and to streamline the methods to enable going faster in places where a learner is outstanding. Here's a math example. Some types of math problems can be solved without doing anything other than applying common sense. I often see such opportunities associ-

Lesson Twenty-One: Adjust the Skill-Learning Method

ated with graphs of equations. If you understand how the signs of variables and constants affect the location and shape of the lines on a graph, by just glancing at an equation you might be able to see a mental image that would be quite close to what could be accurately drawn. If the question related to something like in what quadrants of the standard x-y axis the line falls, nothing more might need be done for such an individual. At the other extreme, some people would have to answer the same question much like someone might apply a paint-by-the-numbers kit (a foolproof way for someone with little talent for painting to produce something better than a disaster). Doing so would mean breaking the task down into many fine chunks, with plenty of directions so that few would get lost or make an error. Think of doing so as being like having a GPS for solving a math problem.

Next, let's consider two people learning to drive a vehicle. One person feels overconfident, drives too fast, and tailgates (drives too close to the vehicle ahead). The other person is fearful, practically leaves the road to avoid being anywhere near the center of a two-lane road, and drives so slowly that drivers are always honking their horns, tailgating, and passing in dangerous ways. Notice that each person needs to focus on quite different practices if their driving skills are to eventually develop to a similar level. With the first person, we need to create more awareness of driving safely. For the second person, we need to create awareness of how a driver's cautious behavior can increase danger. With the first driver, we might practice only where speeding would be impossible due to heavy traffic. For the second driver, we might, instead, practice on mostly unoccupied roads.

Finally, let's look at two learners who are identical in talents, but who are quite different in how they assess their own performance. The first learner only notices his mistakes. He's greatly upset whenever one occurs. He is so affected by being upset that after the first mistake he starts making mistakes that he wouldn't normally make. We need to shift his focus to the idea of making no more than a certain number of relatively harmless mistakes ... and totally avoiding serious mistakes. By contrast, a second learner has a low opinion of her abilities. Consequently, she's unsure whether she's right. As a result, she checks her work a dozen times before moving on. This excessive checking doesn't make her any more accurate than if she performed only one or two appropriate checks. We need to shift her perspective to employing the best ways to check and being satisfied with the results.

I'm sure by now I've convinced you that skill-learning methods will need significant adjustments for each individual. Your learners will thank you for applying this lesson as thoroughly as you can.

Your Assignments

1. How can you use measurements to identify where the skill-learning method needs to be adjusted?

2. How can you then measure how well the adjustments are working?

3. What does the student think is happening?

4. How does the student feel at each point in the learning process?

5. How can the learning process be adjusted to reflect the learner's unique skills and challenges?

6. How does the learning process need to be adjusted to reflect the person's self-image and personality?

7. How can the skill-learning process be changed to instill better habits, ones that are quite different from what the learner usually does?

Lesson Twenty-Two:

Demonstrate Application of the Discipline to Goals

*"If you had known Me,
you would have known My Father also;
and from now on you know Him
and have seen Him."*

*Philip said to Him,
"Lord, show us the Father,
and it is sufficient for us."*

*Jesus said to him,
"Have I been with you so long,
and yet you have not known Me, Philip?*

*He who has seen Me has seen the Father;
so how can you say, 'Show us the Father'?*

*Do you not believe that I am in the Father,
and the Father in Me?*

Lesson Twenty-Two: Demonstrate Application of the Discipline to Goals

> *The words that I speak to you*
> *I do not speak on My own authority;*
> *but the Father who dwells in Me does the works.*
>
> *Believe Me that I am in the Father*
> *and the Father in Me, or else*
> *believe Me for the sake of the works themselves."*
>
> — John 14:7-11 (NKJV)

Many people who are totally confused about how to conduct a discipline's process for accomplishing their goals will actually tell you that they completely understand what to do. You might receive such assurance from a student who wants to please you. Or a student who has a good conceptual grasp of a discipline might tell you so, but the student might still lack a practical sense of how to apply the most important parts of the process. Alternately, the student may have memorized what a number of other people have done to apply the discipline, but that information might not be relevant to accomplishing the student's own goals.

How will you know that such confusion exists? After receiving such lip service, a moment may arise when you say or do something that a student responds to with a question or challenge that indicates her or his source of confusion. We can see such an example of Philip not understanding that Jesus, as God's Son, was the living embodiment of our Heavenly Father.

To deal with Philip's misunderstanding, Jesus explained in two ways that Philip could potentially appreciate: Take Jesus at His word that He was in the Father and the Father was in Him, and consider that the miracles could not have been done without the power and authority of our Heavenly Father. Notice, too, that by explaining in this way Jesus was inviting Philip to know Him better, to fully appreciate His uniqueness.

Likewise, we can expect that some misunderstandings will occur about how to apply a discipline's process, even after effectively demonstrating how to do so for a learner's own goals. Nevertheless, such demonstrations are extremely valuable for creating a learning platform, much as Jesus did by pointing out His miracles to Philip as a way of explaining His connection to our Heavenly Father.

Since you have already applied this discipline to meet your own goals, you will probably find that demonstrating how to apply the discipline to meet the learner's goals will be one of the easier and more effective tasks that you will undertake while teaching breakthrough learning.

However, your initial reaction to doing so may not be as positive. You might be remembering how long it took you to develop your own application of a discipline. Relax. You don't have to duplicate that work to effectively demonstrate an application to your student's goals. I hope that observation makes you feel more encouraged.

Such a demonstration can be accomplished in three ways. First, you can simply find some well-done published work related to the student's goals and draw enough details from the work to describe the steps that were taken. While doing so, you don't have to explain everything. You just need to illustrate each of the significant tasks in some relevant way.

Second, if no such complete example exists, you could piece together parts of relevant examples to demonstrate what the learner needs to appreciate. For such an approach to be most effective, it's helpful to use a partially described example related to the learner's goals as the context for then demonstrating whatever elements are missing from that example. In such a case, you might be able to use detailed, but unrelated, examples to then explain how to do various specific steps by putting that information in the context of the overall example.

Third, should there be no partial example related to the learner's goals, you might construct a completely hypothetical example that contains simulated data. While doing so might appear to be more

Lesson Twenty-Two: Demonstrate Application of the Discipline to Goals

work than engaging in either of the first two alternatives, I've usually found that such an approach can be faster and easier than dealing with real examples. In taking this approach, feel free to customize any templates from your own application by simply inserting simulated data.

However, the main advantage I've found from using such hypothetical examples is that they are simpler, cleaner, and easier for students to follow. By having the freedom to describe and illustrate the demonstration any way you want, you'll probably make the material more transparent, simply because your focus will be on putting together a good demonstration, rather than on actually representing the process that someone else did.

Let me now describe a little about how I usually conduct such demonstrations. I begin by reiterating the student's goals. Although you would think that such goals would already be quite clear to and memorable for students, my experience has sometimes been different. Some students shift their focus and may actually be thinking about doing something different, something even potentially unrelated to what you have prepared, by the time you demonstrate. For instance, such a shift can occur because your prior teaching has introduced an idea or opportunity that powerfully energized the student's imagination. Keep in mind that although a student may have altered focus, he or she may still be interested in seeing a demonstration related to what was once highly relevant to her or him. However, if the goals have changed, check before doing so.

From there, I list the strengths and weaknesses of the discipline as it applies to meeting the student's goals. I try to use precise definitions of these characterizations in terms of the approach I will be demonstrating.

After that, I show a visual that connects and generally describes all of the steps involved in the approach. From then on, I will remind my student where each step fits in the whole process.

In demonstrating each step, I take into account what the student already knows. For instance, if my student has graduate-level knowledge of math, I won't demonstrate the mathematical elements in detail. Instead, I'll just list what the elements are. If, instead, the student is weak in math, I might spell out all of the key elements in a fair amount of detail, using real or simulated values.

Depending on the student's perspective, I will usually begin explaining a step by either showing the output or detailing the aspects of the step in their optimal sequence. Leaders tend not to be interested in the details until after they've seen what the details can do for them. So for someone with such an orientation, I would begin with the output. For someone who is more focused on processes, I would leave sharing the output until after the aspects of the step have been demonstrated.

People vary in how they like information to be formatted. Over the years, I've often put together demonstrations for senior executives showing how their decisions might affect the value of a company's stock. Financial people usually liked to see exhibits that look much like profit-and-loss statements. Operations staffers often preferred exhibits that emphasized the equations used to determine the values. Marketing executives frequently preferred bar graphs and pie charts. The CEOs were often interested in information that could be used to easily calculate the effect on her or his net worth in terms of shares owned and stock options granted. So, be prepared to adjust the way you express the demonstration to a format that will seem most relevant and easy for the student to understand.

Such a demonstration can often be made more compelling by enabling the student to interact with the examples. For instance, if part of the process involves applying equations, you might make those explicit and let the student see some examples with different values in the equations. From examining such information, a student may be able to develop an intuition for what kinds of results will be most valuable for different purposes. Gaining such insights will usually increase interest in applying this process, a useful outcome to result from providing such a demonstration.

Lesson Twenty-Two: Demonstrate Application of the Discipline to Goals

Naturally, if some aspects of the process will be performed by others so that the student doesn't need to know all the details, you can vary that part of the demonstration to focus on just the interaction that should occur with suppliers, staff, or volunteers who will be performing such tasks. If the student will need to select the proper people to do the work, you could certainly include some relevant examples of what information to gather and how to assess it.

One of the hard-won lessons I have gained from delivering such demonstrations is that most people aren't very interested in seeing a demonstration of a discipline ... even when connected to their own goals. Consequently, it will be easy for you to provide more information, in greater detail, and with more complexity than your student is prepared to absorb. When you make such a mistake, the result can be to kill all interest in applying the process to the learner's goals. Why? Well, such a demonstration can make applying a process appear to the student to be like climbing Mount Everest without the proper gear and help, suggesting the likelihood of any attempt to do so ending in a dangerous and painful fiasco.

As a result, I suggest that you make the demonstration quite a bit simpler and shorter than what you think your student would like. However, feel free to prepare intriguing bits and pieces of added information that you can share with a student who seems genuinely enthused to learn more about a given step or aspect. In doing so, you should expect that you'll only have the opportunity to share less than 10 percent of any such supplementary information. So, if appropriate, be comfortable leaving out *all* that supplementary information!

What else might you do to avoid providing too much information, detail, and complexity? Ask the student what he or she would like to see before you put together the demonstration. By doing so, you'll be able to focus the information and detail where a student will find such provision to be desirable, thereby increasing attention and interest as you develop those points. In this way, you'll increase the student's confidence that she or he can succeed in applying the discipline's process by helping to remove any feelings of self-doubt and of being overwhelmed by the required work.

Finally, it's helpful to address what the student may not want to raise directly: What can go wrong and what are the consequences? In most well-designed processes, the risks are usually well contained. Where a student might imagine that making a mistake would lead to doing something harmful, you should be prepared to demonstrate how such a horrible result can be avoided. If the student only learns this one point, then the whole demonstration will be worthwhile. This student probably won't make that kind of error!

Your Assignments

1. What would the student most like to learn about the discipline's application of what you are going to demonstrate?

2. What is the most detail that this student is likely to tolerate?

3. How much detail is the least that's acceptable for this student?

4. Where, if at all, would the student most like to interact with the details?

5. What formats for expressing the information will seem most relevant and be easiest for the student to understand?

6. How long should such a demonstration last?

7. What would make the demonstration a great help to the student for increasing confidence and understanding?

8. What would make such a demonstration a flop for this student?

Lesson Twenty-Three:

Watch and Correct the Learner's Application

He who planted the ear, shall He not hear?
He who formed the eye, shall He not see?
He who instructs the nations, shall He not correct,
He who teaches man knowledge?
The LORD knows the thoughts of man,
That they are *futile.*
Blessed is *the man whom You instruct, O LORD,*
And teach out of Your law,
That You may give him rest from the days of adversity,
Until the pit is dug for the wicked.

— Psalm 94:9-13 (NKJV)

Regardless of a student's skill, expertise, knowledge, confidence, and desire, he or she will make at least some mistakes in applying a discipline to succeed with goals. As Psalm 94:9-13 (NKJV) reminds us, those who are applying any futile thoughts or making any wrong actions need to be redirected by God. Since you and I cannot hope to approach anywhere near God's knowledge and understanding, that realization should encourage us to seek direction from God through His Holy Spirit for teaching our students. By then following such direction, our students will receive better help from us.

Lesson Twenty-Three: Watch and Correct the Learner's Application

Let's begin this lesson by discussing how to watch what a student does. Naturally, there are limits to what merely watching can tell us. Unless you happen to be a mind reader, watching is not one of the best ways to understand what a student is thinking. Consequently, I find it helpful to gain more information from the student before beginning to watch.

Let me explain with a purposely extreme example. Imagine that a student incorrectly believes that by jumping off a tall cliff he or she will draw closer to God by provoking Him to provide a miraculous rescue. We know that doing so is based on a false belief; Jesus pointed out in Matthew 4:7 (NKJV) that we are not to tempt God in this way, quoting Deuteronomy 6:16 (NKJV). If I only watch such a student, I might merely observe the horror of a fatal jump ... providing no benefit to the student. If, instead, I first ask the student to tell me what she or he plans to do, I can point out to the student why the jump is not a good idea, hopefully preventing his or her immediate death. May all of our students' mistaken beliefs and plans be less dangerous than my example!

Because of my desire for students to avoid significant mistakes and harm, I always ask for descriptions of a student's plans before anything is done. Reading and discussing step-by-step drafts of plans have always revealed deficiencies in the student's understanding of how best to apply the discipline. Addressing such deficiencies has then helped every student by either reducing errors or saving time.

I then use any indications of confusion, lack of knowledge, or misunderstandings to identify any needs for changes. In communicating my concerns, I avoid dictating an answer. While the student might prefer for me to provide the "right" answer, doing so would eliminate opportunities to identify other ways to help the student. Ironing out the sources of potential problems could require several rounds of drafting by the student, followed by my commenting on such drafts.

Once the overall plan looks to be as good as it can be made by a student, I then ask the student to spell out in even more detail what she or he will do first. After that, the rounds of student drafting, comments by me, and redrafting by the student continue on in the first step.

After the student appears to be on a fruitful track, I will suggest that implementing the first step begin. I will ask the student to keep a detailed journal of what is done and how much time he or she spends daily on each aspect of the step. While it's not the same as watching what the student does, I can use the combination of seeing the results of the first step and reading the journal to get a rough sense of what has gone on. When the first step is complete, I will give the student written comments on both the output and the application of time described in the journal. In the latter case, I will focus on whether the student has spent the right amount of time and in the best ways. As you might expect, the first step might also have to be redone to correct errors.

I will repeat this kind of interaction during each subsequent step, no matter how small. Since I'm usually hundreds or even thousands of miles away from my students, these communications will usually be accomplished by means of e-mail, reviewing written materials and measurements, and occasional Skype conversations. As students complete more steps, they will become far more efficient and effective.

While this description of what I will do might make it seem as if such "watching" always goes smoothly, any smoothness is the exception rather than the rule. One of the main things I will have to be vigilant in watching for is a student who is in trouble ... but who doesn't seek help. The first indication I may receive of such a problem will be silence that lasts too long, which can tip me off that I need to intervene. Having performed activities similar to what my students are doing, I will have a pretty good idea of how long each one should take for the student.

If I don't receive results when they should be done, I will send a gently probing e-mail inquiring about how the work is progressing and how I can help. In return, I will hope to receive an update and an explanation for the delay. Naturally, I will need a response before

Lesson Twenty-Three: Watch and Correct the Learner's Application

I can help. Unfortunately, I often don't receive one. That is a very bad sign; something has caused a substantial problem. It may be an issue at work or at home, but I still won't know what to suggest until I learn what is happening with the student. So I will allow 48 hours to go by, and then I will resend the first message, noting that it must not have been received. In some cases, the e-mail will have disappeared somewhere in cyberspace. However, in most instances, the individual will be so preoccupied with something that has nothing to do with applying the discipline that there will have been either no time or not enough attention available for contacting me. Under such duress, some students will just disappear. However, if that happens to you, don't give up hope. I have had students resurface as many as seven years later, acting as if nothing had happened. When that occurs, I usually learn that a severe problem had arisen, such as illness of a parent, death of a spouse, loss of a job, or difficulties at work that took all of the person's extra time and energy.

When I receive reports or can directly observe the student, I have to be equally aware of what isn't being said or done. For example, while students may have understood all of what was required at an intellectual level, they may have decided to initially focus their attention on just part of performing a step. In doing so, it's not uncommon for them to forget that there are other tasks to be done. In their eagerness to complete the work, they may not go back and perform those other parts until I remind them.

In fact, there's a specially challenging subcategory of such students that I too often meet: ones who never seem to be able to keep the instructions for what to do next. No matter how many times I send directions, these students come back a few days later asking questions about what to do, questions that were thoroughly covered in the instructions they had already received. What does such an interaction mean? In most cases, I have found that I am dealing with an individual who is strongly affected by some harmful habit or disability that blocks or delays making efficient progress. Although I may never know what the habit or disability is, I can only try to help by being patient, sending the relevant information again, and gently pointing out that it had been previously sent.

Okay, let's assume you have gotten past such problems. What should you look for in reviewing what a student has done or is doing? *I suggest you look into everything.* Why? Otherwise, you could easily miss opportunities to help a student improve. For instance, that nice PowerPoint presentation with the neat exhibits and clear focus may be based on calculation errors or misunderstanding what kind of analysis was required.

So be sure to look at the details of how the results were generated. In the process, you may find some big surprises. I learned this lesson the hard way while working with a talented MBA on my consulting firm's staff. He had performed analyses to determine the attractiveness of making various acquisitions for a client. While I was troubled by noticing that each acquisition my colleague had analyzed seemed to be very appealing, I failed to investigate why that was so. Only after presenting the results to the client did I learn that the MBA had made an incorrect assumption in his calculations: He believed that the purchaser of a company didn't have to pay back any money that the acquired company had already borrowed. Wrong! Needless to say, I ate some humble pie that day, apologized, and asked to come back with the results of the correct calculations. Fortunately, the client forgave us, and we were able to accurately complete the work.

Also, check to see that the transfer of the work product into the exhibits has been done correctly. It is easy for students to become confused about what numbers or kinds of information are relevant to their exhibits. In such cases, a student may have the right information, but not include it in the exhibits.

Proper sequencing of information development is often hard for students to accomplish. If you can't follow a line of logic from the information provided, be sure to ask questions about any gaps. It may well be that the student skipped a step.

Lesson Twenty-Three: Watch and Correct the Learner's Application

If I seem to be directing you to look everywhere, then you are correctly remembering my advice. Let me use an analogy to explain why doing so is important. Imagine that you are a firefighter called to a scene where there's smoke, but no flames are observable. While it's possible that someone has merely set off a smoke bomb inside a structure, that is unlikely. It is also important to assume that there's a fire somewhere until such time as that possibility can be definitively ruled out.

As you enter the structure, there is no one present to tell you what's going on. Since you haven't been in this particular building before, you don't know where all the rooms are, the way to the basement, and what is stored on the premises. To be safe, you need to be prepared for anything that might come your way. The fire might be in the walls, in the basement below, or even outside one part of the structure. If you don't pay attention, you could, instead, pay with your life or receive a severe injury.

Such vigilance will pay off for you in your role as a teacher, as well. A disastrous risk or error could be anywhere.

As you look critically at the student's work, however, only do so in ways that will *not* convey to the student anything other than confidence in the student's ability to apply the discipline. For instance, while I scan for disastrous errors, I'm usually praising aloud the student's work for anything I notice that has been done acceptably.

Here's one final caution: Don't assume that a student has successfully followed your directions after you've pointed out something that needs correction. Simply because an error has already occurred in some aspect of the work, there's a strong possibility that a student is still confused. Any time you find that such a correction has been made improperly, be sure to vary your subsequent explanations to increase the chances of establishing accurate understanding.

Your Assignments

1. Where is a student most likely to make errors in applying the discipline?

2. What steps can you direct the student to take that will make avoiding errors easier?

3. How can you improve the student's efficiency and effectiveness in doing these tasks?

4. How can you spot more of the errors that have already occurred?

5. What is the best way to help this student correct any errors?

6. How will you help a student who isn't responsive?

Lesson Twenty-Four:

Measure and Address Underlying Causes of Errors and Slowness

You shall have a perfect and just weight,
a perfect and just measure,
that your days may be lengthened in the land
which the Lord your God is giving you.

— Deuteronomy 25:15 (NKJV)

And they shall rebuild the old ruins,
They shall raise up the former desolations,
And they shall repair the ruined cities,
The desolations of many generations.

— Isaiah 61:4 (NKJV)

I've provided this lesson to share what I've learned about the difficulties of correctly identifying and effectively addressing the *underlying causes* of a student's errors and slowness. Think of such causes as being ones that affect the student's performance in a number of steps and tasks. While you can certainly focus solely on helping the student to work more accurately and faster while performing each task,

Lesson Twenty-Four: Measure and Address Underlying Causes of Errors and Slowness

you will make better progress if you also address underlying causes that aren't obvious when looking at an individual instance.

I was reminded of the difficulties in identifying underlying causes just yesterday while driving my wife to the airport. While doing so, I drove under a number of bridges that had been brightly painted in the last two or three years.

Each bridge had looked as if it were brand new when first painted. However, since then the paint has been falling off in big chunks to reveal massive amounts of rust ... so much rust that I wondered if the bridges were about to collapse.

I then speculated about what the underlying causes of so much corrosion might have been. Did the painters fail to scrape off the old rust before painting? Or did they use a paint that didn't sufficiently protect the steel from water? Could the corrosion have been made worse by all the salt put on Boston-area roads during winter storms? Could the bridges have been allowed to rust for so long before being repainted that there was little that could have been done to arrest the latest rusting?

Then, my thoughts shifted to the enormous expense involved in building one of such bridges. When initially constructed, the steel beams look so strong and pristine, as though they might last forever. Clearly, perfection had been the initial objective. However, once the bridges were put into use, perfection no longer seemed to have been the goal. Presumably a different set of people were in charge at that point. Did they earn bonuses for underspending on maintenance by doing less painting than would have been desirable? It's possible.

Next, I thought about how the road is operated. The Massachusetts Turnpike is managed by the same governmental authority that was in charge of the so-called Big Dig in Boston, a project that added two new harbor tunnels, replaced a major surface highway with a new road beneath the city, and added a bridge to the north. While initially planned to cost $2.8 billion, the expenditures escalated to over $14 billion. Due to these enormous cost overruns, maintenance might have been cut on the existing roads, including the part I was driving on. Perhaps the decision to do such a large project without fully understanding the underground situation was the true underlying cause of those pitiful-looking bridge beams, so wretchedly exposed as my wife and I whizzed beneath them.

Have I actually measured anything about these bridges that could identify underlying causes? No, of course, I haven't. All I've done is list some of the thoughts that might lead me to make measurements that could potentially reveal the actual cause or causes.

Why then did I share these thoughts? Well, I wanted you to appreciate that most people would at this point simply take one of the thoughts and decide that it was the cause ... and then proceed to deal with the situation accordingly. As you can imagine, the chances of fixing the problem in this way are slim, at best.

When we merely go with our own judgments about causes of any slowness and errors based on no measurements, we are making a subjective decision, which if it favors our own interests would be similar to using dishonest measures and weights when selling products to others ... something that is not approved of by God, as evidenced by Deuteronomy 25:15 (NKJV). To gain the long life promised in that verse, we need to, instead, always apply objective, honest measures.

What should be done, instead? In the case of these bridges, we might initially read any recommendations that the original engineers made about maintenance, find out what type of paint was previously applied, determine what the effectiveness of such paint should have been, look into how often repainting should have occurred, and examine any photographs of doing such work. I have not looked for that information, but most of it is probably available in some form or other. By doing so I might be able to determine that either the maintenance had been done adequately and the corrosion was unavoidable ... or that the maintenance was faulty. If the latter, I should find out if the decision of what and when to do maintenance was at fault, or if the work was done incorrectly.

Lesson Twenty-Four: Measure and Address Underlying Causes of Errors and Slowness

If the maintenance had been poorly performed, I would next need to measure the training that preceded the work. If these methods were flawed, I should then see who decided to use them. And so on.

If the work had been done correctly, but long after it would be have timely, then I will need to determine why the decisions to delay were made. I might find some connection to incentives for delaying maintenance, the maintenance staff failing to recommend that the work be done, or possibly even some illegality, such as stealing paint.

If the delay was unavoidable due to budget constraints, then I would look into any possible connection to the Big Dig and its huge cost overruns. And so on.

As I'm sure you can now appreciate, using measurements to find the underlying cause or causes of an occurrence can involve quite a lot of digging, most of which won't do more than rule out some of the many possibilities. However, in working with a student, you can do better in searching for underlying causes because of having the plans of what the student intended to do, as well as the results. Consequently, you should mostly think about what such information tells you, rather than doing a lot of digging to get other information ... of the sort required by my bridge example.

From the plans and results, you'll develop some ideas about what might have gone wrong. Once you have some hypotheses in hand about the causes of slowness and errors, you can then ask your student to tell you more about what she or he did and explain why he or she acted in such ways. In my experience, such questioning will reveal useful answers to about one-third of what has been going on. So that's a good start.

But where can you find answers for the other two-thirds of what has been happening? Well, have the student repeat the tasks while you closely observe. For instance, instead of looking at just the output of a student's step, you should watch while the work is done that created the incorrect output. Hopefully, the student will have retained some notes or work product so that duplicating what was done won't require much added effort for him or her.

If for some reason it would be too time consuming, difficult, or expensive to repeat the work, you can, instead, ask the student to walk you through what was done by asking detailed questions about where data came from, what was done with the data, what the student remembers about how the results looked at various points, the ways results were turned into the final format, and so forth. In doing so, become more detailed while exploring those aspects where you suspect a student was most likely to have made an error. Apply your own experience as well as your knowledge of the student to determine where to look more closely.

So what should you be looking for through such questioning and watching? I suggest that you pay the most attention to anything that seems like it is or could be connected to a pattern. Let me explain by sharing an example. I just reviewed the test results of a student who got the lowest score I have ever seen on a certain kind of standardized test. In fact, the score was so low that random guessing should have provided a higher number of correct answers. Now, this person seems perfectly intelligent. So what might be going on?

First, I checked to see if consecutive answers were off in a way that indicated having made a mistake on the scoring sheet, such as would occur by skipping a question and forgetting to leave a corresponding answer space blank while doing so. That wasn't it. Second, I looked at the questions and the answers the student selected. Here, I found two clues. The chosen answers were almost all off the topic of the questions. Such a result could only occur due to some fundamental misunderstanding of what was being asked. Next, I noticed that in many cases the selected answer was one that repeated a word from the text that was the subject of the question. Now, in many schools and standardized tests, repeating a word from the text is often intended by the test makers as a clue to finding the correct answer. It occurred to me that this student might have been applying such an approach for at least part of the time. Third, I then checked another section of the test that included similar kinds of questions. Here, the student did much better, but still poorly. From looking at these other answers, it occurred to me that the student might have done the two sections on different days. If the student had graded the results from the first section before starting the second one, seeing those answers and explanations could have informed the student in a way that enabled some learning to occur. If so, it may well be that this student can quickly learn after being introduced to better methods.

I'll find out for sure when we meet to review the results. I'll ask for explanations then for why each of the incorrect answers was selected. As I do, I'll pay especially close attention to any universal, underlying misunderstandings about what is being asked and how to answer such questions. In light of such poor results, it's quite likely that this student has several such misunderstandings.

Here's another example of looking for a pattern. A student performed brilliantly on all the hardest material but was hopelessly inept on the easy questions. As I studied the results, I began to realize that there was a pattern. The student was always choosing an answer that could have been connected to the text, if you used quite a bit of imagination. However, if you read the text quite literally, there were no explicit or implicit connections to the chosen answers. After seeing this, I concluded that the student normally worked in a field that rewarded making imaginative, lateral connections, such as English literature or history. Well, the student turned out to be a history major. Having been one myself, I then explained the difference between historical analysis using analogies and what was being asked on this test. Within three hours, the student understood the point and went on to perform nearly flawlessly in the easy portions of the test, as well.

I've been addressing patterns of errors so far in these two examples. What about slowness? The underlying causes of it are usually easier to identify. We previously reviewed one common cause: excessive checking. Another frequent cause can be choosing a complicated method, rather than taking reasonable shortcuts where those will almost always be accurate and routine checking can easily find any erroneous results. Working slowly on purpose is also a likely cause. Some students will do so thinking that working slower makes them more accurate. However, doing so usually doesn't help accuracy unless a student was previously trying to go too fast. While going too slowly, students' attention often wanders, which will always reduce accuracy. In many instances of slowness, some other unneeded steps are being taken and need to be eliminated, such as having others be involved where they add little or no value. Finally, slowness can simply be related to not having done enough of the right kind of practice.

What if you don't see any underlying causes of errors and slowness? Be skeptical of concluding that there are none. Such would only be true if a student were performing near perfectly. If the student's results are below the 99th percentile for effectiveness, then there is bound to be at least one underlying cause that needs to be addressed.

In all of these activities, keep in mind the wisdom expressed in Isaiah 61:4 (NKJV). If the student has been doing the wrong things for a long time, then improving on those beliefs, habits, and practices may be quite a bit like repairing desolated buildings that have been deteriorating for many generations. In fact, your students may actually be repeating ineffective and harmful actions that their parents and grandparents favored, used, and taught them. Be patient as you work with a student on making changes, realizing that Rome wasn't built in a day.

Your Assignments:

1. Where are error rates excessive?

2. Where is there unusual slowness?

Lesson Twenty-Four: Measure and Address Underlying Causes of Errors and Slowness

3. What's different about the results where there are either excessive error rates or unusual slowness?

4. What's different about what the student does during those activities?

5. What are the possible common factors that could be accounting for such errors and slowness?

6. How can speaking with the student rule in or rule out some of those possibilities?

7. What can be learned by directly observing the student doing some of the activities that might be affected by common underlying causes?

8. How should such observations be conducted?

9. How can the student be most effectively helped to change practices?

Lesson Twenty-Five:

Direct the Learner to Self-Improve the Process

*For it is better, if it is the will of God,
to suffer for doing good than for doing evil.*

— 1 Peter 3:17 (NKJV)

1 Peter 3:17 (NKJV) points out that when it is God's will that we suffer for having done a good thing, such suffering is far superior to any suffering that results from our own sinning. In the former case, we can have peace by knowing that God has a purpose for our suffering, a peace that softens the suffering's sting. In the latter instance, we know that we have brought the suffering on ourselves, which can increase the pain.

However, I believe that God will rarely intend for you or your student to suffer while the student self-improves a discipline's process. Consequently, this lesson emphasizes ways to avoid any unnecessary suffering caused by human decisions while doing so.

You might have found self-improving a process to have been one of the most difficult parts of your own breakthrough learning. Your initial concerns about being able to do so may have been even greater than the difficulties you eventually overcame. Keep those perspectives in mind as you direct learners to self-improve a process for accomplishing their goals.

Lesson Twenty-Five: Direct the Learner to Self-Improve the Process

Start by remembering all of the reasons why you were initially concerned either that you wouldn't be able to self-improve a process or that doing so would be more difficult than it actually turned out to be. Your learners are likely to be having some of the same unnecessary concerns.

A good way to diffuse any anxiety related to false concerns is by sharing your own experiences with being concerned and then describing how the reality turned out to be better than you had expected. While doing so, encourage students to share their concerns. If these issues arose during your earlier improvement activities, share your experiences and the lessons you learned from them. To the extent that the student's challenges will be similar, point that out. If the student's task will be more difficult in some ways, describe some methods for reducing at least portions of the unavoidable difficulty.

Realize and explain that while the student's task may be more difficult than yours, sharing your knowledge and experience will reduce the challenges by redirecting the student's concerns to those areas where being careful can be the most helpful. Where the student's task will be easier than yours was, point out that encouraging information, as well.

You probably wasted some time while making your own process improvements. Tell your student what you did that wasted time and then explain how such errors could be reduced or eliminated by her or him. If the student removes any unnecessary activities, you'll actually be reducing the size of the task.

Students vary quite a great deal in the boldness with which they tackle self-improving a process. Some will want to do the minimum, in the least stressful way. Others will want to achieve the maximum, and they won't mind doing lots of challenging work to get there. Much of the difference will relate to the amount of passion the student has for achieving the goals.

For the more timid, you might suggest a narrower scope of inquiry. For instance, you could point out that among the examples of applying the process there were differences in practices that might be combined for the first time. In doing so, be sure to point out what those differences are and to suggest a few ways to combine them. By having scoped out a process-improvement starting point in this way, the student can then focus on avoiding errors and slowness in combining such process elements.

If such an opportunity for combining practices doesn't appear to exist, but there are many other process examples that have not yet been examined, you could suggest that the student scan a reasonable sample of such processes from different kinds of applications to look for optional practices. If doing so seems like too much work for this student, suggest, instead, contacting disciplinary experts who might be able to point to useful examples of optional practices. Such trawling for possibilities might turn up opportunities for new, compatible combinations of practices.

Let's now turn to the bold student. Someone who wants to accomplish the most can be aided in two possible ways:

1. Simultaneously looking in all the highest potential areas
2. Applying a breakthrough method such as 2,000 percent solutions, complementary 2,000 percent solutions, or excellent solutions

Of course, someone who is unusually motivated and energetic could certainly use both approaches. However, for purposes of simplifying our discussion, let me separately treat the two.

How might the student identify what are the best potential areas? While a number of approaches could turn out to be fruitful, I suggest that any believing students begin with prayer seeking guidance from the Holy Spirit and to be refilled with the Holy Spirit. I'm reminded of the importance of doing so by an experience with prayer I had just last night. In preparing to start my next book, I feel even more unprepared and inadequate than usual, which is saying a lot about my concerns. Within five minutes of the prayer, my mind was filled with the most wonderful concepts and methods for accomplishing this task. Please appreciate that I could have worked on

Lesson Twenty-Five: Direct the Learner to Self-Improve the Process

this problem by myself for the rest of my life and not come up with anything nearly as good as what I received in response to this prayer.

After gaining such Godly insights, there will still be ways to use mere human reason and common sense to identify other opportunities. Let's consider next how the student should think about what are the highest potential places for process improvements. Students should start by looking at what took the most time. Surely, there can be ways to reduce the delays, or even just the amount of effort required. Sometimes doing so can be as simple as being more careful in determining how much accuracy is needed for the answer. Since developing more precise answers is much slower and takes more effort, such an adjustment can be a simple solution. Another possibility is involving those who have more access to information or more skill to do the most time-consuming tasks. I've often benefitted from obtaining the output from someone's database in only a few days and avoided months of tedious work by so doing. Finding such alternatives normally requires some looking. As I have mentioned before, speaking with those who are experts in the discipline might lead your student to such sources. Also, students should look at published materials to see if they credit any unique sources. If your students find any such references, they should be sure to contact those who are credited to find out what they or their organizations can do for your student's application of the process.

A parallel search can be conducted that focuses, instead, on those aspects of the process where errors have most often occurred. In this instance, the student should be looking for methods that will avoid many of the most common sources of errors, and will be simpler and easier to do.

Most processes also have too many steps. It can be quite helpful to set some arbitrary goal for how many steps the process should have, such as half the number of steps, and then consider how such a reduction might be accomplished. Seeking to make such a substantial change is helpful because it will require the student to approach the process from a totally new perspective.

Here's an example. Prior to Mitchell and Company developing its proprietary process for identifying the likely stock-price effects of making a series of major changes, analysts almost always looked at such changes in isolation from one another. Because the amount of work involved in analyzing every change was so substantial, most companies only considered a few of them. Our firm took the approach of wanting to increase how many changes could be considered and in how many different sequences. As a consequence of setting that goal, the number of steps involved in the process was reduced by billions of times so that what was once considered impractical became quite easy to accomplish in a short amount of time. The key was designing a screening step that would be low cost and quick to eliminate all but a handful of combined, high-potential choices. This result was accomplished by conducting anonymously sponsored interviews of current and potential shareholders to find the few actions that would cause them to buy or sell significant amounts of stock. No one else had apparently added such a step to the process. Consequently, focus was placed on many fewer, and more valuable, combinations and sequences of changes.

As you can see from this example, it's helpful to look for places where processes are being repeated sequentially for solving pieces of the puzzle. Then ask this question: How can the whole puzzle be solved in just one application of the process?

While I could go on to add other examples, let me switch, instead, to the subject of teaching a student one of the powerful problem-solving methods, such as how to develop excellent solutions, complementary 2,000 percent solutions, or 2,000 percent solutions. Of course, determining which process to use is related to how big an improvement the student wants to make. Without a huge improvement goal, there may be no need for applying anything more than the 2,000 percent solution process, which can reduce the time, money, and effort involved in a process by 96 percent or more from implementing one solution. The same process can also be used to reduce errors by a similar amount.

Lesson Twenty-Five: Direct the Learner to Self-Improve the Process

While a student can certainly decide to replace the whole process using one of these three breakthrough methods, be sure that your student is aware that any of these methods can also be applied to a single aspect or just a few aspects of the existing process. Doing so will naturally be much easier to accomplish than replacing almost all of the steps of the process the student just used. Working on that specific aspect might also match some frustration that the student felt while applying the process, thus increasing motivation.

Here's an example. While I was in college, I worked part-time at the alumni magazine. My job primarily related to updating the mailing list to be sure that the magazines were sent to the right address. While that sounds easy to do, it was somewhat complicated by the fact that some alumni owned so many homes that they might live in seven or eight of them during a single year, and not follow any particular pattern as to when they did so. Also, we received notices of address changes from many different sources, some of which lagged the others by several months. So there was a guessing game involved to some extent in figuring out what was the best address to use for someone who was quickly shifting from one temporary location to another.

Having done this work for three years, I knew all about the ways that the process worked poorly, took too long, and was frustrating to apply. When the publisher of the magazine asked me to help lead the development of a better process, I was ready to go. As a result, we were able to scrap almost all of the time-consuming and error-inducing elements of the old process.

However, I suspect that the student's first application of a process will have operated much better than did this magazine's way of updating mailing addresses, so there won't usually be as much frustration to fire imagination for making improvements. Be sure to focus on helping the student tap into whatever frustration is felt.

Of course, many students will fall between the extremes of wanting to do the least and the most. For helping them decide how to proceed, you should begin by describing how to perform the two extremes. Doing so might help shift a middling focus into a different one, simply by appealing to some aspect of what a student is curious about or is frustrated by. When that happens, you'll soon begin receiving questions about how to tackle other kinds of process self-improvements. Answer those questions in such a way that the student can compare alternatives and make a wise decision about which approach to apply for self-improving the process.

Your Assignments

1. What frustrated the student about conducting the process?

2. What would the student most like to change about the process?

3. How committed is the student to making small versus large improvements?

4. How capable is the student of learning a breakthrough-improvement process?

5. How does the student respond to your descriptions of various ways to self-improve the process?

6. What methods of self-improving the process are most likely to be fruitful and rewarding for this student?

7. Have can the student be directed to engage in this activity so that errors and delays will be avoided?

Lesson Twenty-Six:

Demonstrate How to Update Information and Knowledge

"Do not remember the former things,
Nor consider the things of old.
Behold, I will do a new thing,
Now it shall spring forth;
Shall you not know it?
I will even make a road in the wilderness
And rivers in the desert.
The beast of the field will honor Me,
The jackals and the ostriches,
Because I give waters in the wilderness
And rivers in the desert,
To give drink to My people, My chosen.
This people I have formed for Myself;
They shall declare My praise."

— Isaiah 43:18-21 (NKJV)

Isaiah 43:18-21 (NKJV) reminds us to keep expecting God to provide new and improved conditions. While many followers of Jesus equate this reference to Jesus' second coming, these verses can also be read more broadly to apply to the potential for God to enhance His provision for us before then.

Lesson Twenty-Six: Demonstrate How to Update Information and Knowledge

Regardless of whether the second interpretation is valid, I remain an optimist because of having been rewarded again and again by believing that God would miraculously make a better way for others, as well as for me. Such optimism also means that I am deeply convinced that God is capable and willing to provide me with some new information and knowledge that will make what now exists seem like a mere grain of sand on a beach compared to what is to come.

For instance, when starting The 400 Year Project in 1995, I had no clue for how I could ever play a contributing role for fulfilling that project's goal: identifying and demonstrating how 400 years of normal improvements could be implemented in only 20 years from 2015 through 2035. Yet, by 2014, God had disclosed to me three remarkable methods that would make such an accomplishment possible, culminating in excellent solutions that enable making hundreds of thousands of years' worth of normal improvements in one set of changes that would take less than a year to accomplish. What was the difference that enabled so much more to be done? God provided something new that was astoundingly better.

Now, since God is all-knowing, He was always aware of this better way. Why hadn't it been provided before? I don't know, but perhaps He intended someone else to first describe and apply this process, but that person did not listen. For instance, His provision could have been ignored by someone who should have been seeking to update information and knowledge about how to do more for expanding and improving God's Kingdom. Perhaps several such people ignored God's message. Perhaps He's been sending this knowledge for thousands of years and everyone ignored it. Or, perhaps God provided this knowledge now because of some special plans He has for the immediate years to come.

In this lesson, I encourage you to first describe for your students how God has answered your prayers for being more fruitful in applying breakthrough learning, including ways of learning new information and knowledge. First, share what some of those prayers have been. Second, describe why you think that God might have answered the prayers that He did. Third, tell what a difference God's provision made. Fourth, discuss your students' ideas about how they might approach God in prayer to humbly seek His amazing support. By doing so, you might help your students draw closer to Jesus in ways that would not have occurred as much or as soon. When that happens, every aspect of your students' activities can become much more fruitful.

After having accomplished these four tasks, I urge you then to continue helping your students by describing your experiences with keeping up-to-date on information and knowledge from any Earthly sources. While exhortations to conduct such tracking and applying of what is learned can seem quite empty to learners, practical examples of what you have accomplished by doing so will make this activity seem work seem much more relevant and compelling.

One of the best ways to increase the impact of what you share is by describing the consequences of what would probably have happened had you not updated your information and knowledge from Earthly sources. I suggest focusing on the examples where the differences in possible consequences were greatest.

Here's an example from my own experiences. Like most other people in the world, I once thought that you didn't need to talk to investors to identify a company's best decisions for improving stock price. I not only believed in this position, but I also argued in favor of my position with anyone who would listen.

Then, one day the investor-relations executive for a very large company told me that he was willing to spend his company's money to prove me wrong and to teach me an important lesson I needed to learn. Well, how could I resist such an offer? Now, I appreciate that God must surely have been inspiring this man's generous offer, but at the time I didn't perceive that connection.

The results of the interviews we conducted stunned me. Almost all of the company's largest shareholders believed that the company would implement eight favorably viewed actions in the following year, none of which the executives intended to do. As we discussed

Lesson Twenty-Six: Demonstrate How to Update Information and Knowledge

what this information might mean, the conclusion was obvious: If this company did not do most of those actions, many shareholders were going to be unhappy, and at least some of them would sell their positions in disgust. No one at the client company wanted such a result to occur. Consequently, the leaders adjusted their plans to reflect the wisdom behind some of the actions that large investors preferred and expected. Many billions of dollars in shareholder investments were probably saved in the process (at least in the near term), and my firm was launched into learning how to use a powerful new method for identifying optimal ways to enhance and sustain a public company's share price. In the process, I had added the keystone for eventually creating the successful consulting practice that provided almost all of my company's revenues and profits for many years to come. Thank you, Lord!

As happened in this last example, sometimes new information can just fall into your lap. Encourage your students to be open to gaining such help by expending whatever added effort or expense is required. Be sure to point out that humble sources requiring little time and attention can often be quite useful.

Here's an example. I experienced a valuable form of such updating today. I had been struck in recent years that there had not been as much innovation in the business models of what for-profit social enterprises (ones that place at least as much emphasis on improving society as they do on earning profits) do as would be desirable for those who are sincere in accomplishing a social mission. After closing my e-mail account, I happened to see a teaser for a five-minute video about a relatively new company that provides products to help women keep their underwear clean during menstruation, and after having lost some control over urination or elimination. The products aim to be effective, while also giving women more confidence and comfort while in public. Part of the proceeds from certain sales is earmarked to provide free sanitary napkins to girls in underdeveloped nations who might normally stay home from school due to the lack of such items. Portions of other proceeds pay for surgeries in emerging countries to repair the bladders of women who suffered tears during childbirth, protecting them from divorce and ostracism. The firm also uses a supplier who pays its factory workers two-and-a-half times the usual wage to produce these items. By spending just these few moments, I was able to learn and appreciate a great deal about how a more caring and all-encompassing version of a social enterprise could be established. This experience greatly encouraged me to keep updating my information and knowledge in this regard. Wouldn't anyone with similar interests be so encouraged?

From your own experiences with updating knowledge and information and your observations of how your students benefitted from what they have learned while applying their disciplines' processes, you should be able to suggest some of the more effective ways for students to do their own updating. As you consider what advice to provide, take into account ways that a student can be encouraged to take all of the appropriate steps. For instance, what does the student like to do? Can that liking be tied to doing something that would provide useful updates? What does the student hate to do? How can those activities be avoided while updating? Are there any methods that would make such updating occur automatically? What role could incentives play in encouraging the proper actions? For example, could a student who isn't likely to update information and knowledge inexpensively hire someone who would routinely do the work and report just the helpful results? Or is there an existing resource that could be used for this purpose in a way that the student would find interesting and enjoyable?

One possibility you should consider is introducing students to others with similar passions. As a result, they could exchange information that they uncover, thus encouraging one another to keep looking. I have seen such sharing among my students who later encouraged others to study with me. While such referring students did brilliantly in their own work, one reason for their enthusiasm, the students they referred to me did still better. I suspect that the first students helped the referred students to set higher expectations and

Lesson Twenty-Six: Demonstrate How to Update Information and Knowledge

probably shared some helpful lessons for meeting them. I am sure that many such students are doing so informally. As you teach more students, you would be able to expand such connections by bringing people with similar goals together, even if they are focused on different disciplines to accomplish their goals.

Keep in mind that a cautionary example about not staying up-to-date drawn from the discipline can be worth 10,000 reminders to do so. If you know of such an example or could quickly find one, it would be well worth doing so. My experience is that obsolete business processes continue to plod along, often for as long as 100 years after they have been surpassed. Chances are that you can find such anachronisms by simply doing some online word searches concerning long-established organizations and any of their methods that relate to the student's discipline.

I would probably only need to read a summary of the ten newest "hot" books about business management to find at least seven that would be espousing methods that are way out of date. To make the point, I could then compare the results that the authors are touting could be achieved by applying their "hot" methods to what could be accomplished by using any of The 400 Year Project's processes. If you have no other potential comparison to make, I suggest that you follow suit to make this same point. You could also leave the student in anticipatory suspense by simply mentioning that God could reveal a still better breakthrough method that would leave excellent solutions in the dust. If that were to occur, why wouldn't everyone want to use such a much better method?

The point is relevant. Based on the e-mails I receive from students who once worked with me in creating and implementing 2,000 percent solutions, it is obvious that hardly any of them bothered to learn about and apply complementary 2,000 percent solutions. By not staying up-to-date in this way, they missed an opportunity to become 20 times more effective in applying what they had already learned. Of those who worked on complementary 2,000 percent solutions, hardly any have learned about excellent solutions, cutting themselves off from the biggest potential gain they could make from learning anything. Such missed opportunities have occurred despite my doing as much as possible to increase awareness of and encourage learning the improved methods. Don't let your students make these mistakes by becoming complacent about what they know!

Finally, I suggest that you pray for God to increase your students' interest in staying up-to-date on what He provides so that they can increase and improve His Kingdom. In doing so, ask Him to lead you to do anything that He wants done to achieve this purpose.

Your Assignments

1. How can you encourage your students to be highly interested and active in staying aware of valuable new information and knowledge?

2. How can that work be kept as simple as possible?

3. How can the time demands be reduced?

4. How can the updating be made as interesting and enjoyable as possible?

5. How can the costs be reduced to an affordable level?

6. How can the significance of new information and knowledge be most quickly and accurately perceived by the students?

Lesson Twenty-Seven:

Improve Your Teaching by Repeating the Steps for Teaching Others

I have more understanding than all my teachers,
For Your testimonies are *my meditation.*
I understand more than the ancients,
Because I keep Your precepts.

— Psalm 119:99-100 (NKJV)

Psalm 119:99-100 (NKJV) powerfully reminds us that God is our ultimate source of all breakthrough learning. The more we can operate as He does in applying what He directs, the more we will accomplish with teaching and applying such learning.

Let's first focus on some of the ways God operates. He is always available to us through sending our prayers. We need to be accessible to our students, as well.

God is also in all believers, in the form of the Holy Spirit. This embodiment isn't neutral; the Holy Spirit changes us to be more like Jesus. Consequently, our teaching needs to instill better habits that will change how our students spend their time in ways that will increase and improve God's Kingdom.

Lesson Twenty-Seven: Improve Your Teaching by Repeating the Steps for Teaching Others

God also helps those who seek His support for accomplishing His purposes. We need to be similarly helpful to current and past students who want to master applying breakthrough learning.

God wants everyone to choose Salvation. We should be prepared to teach breakthrough learning to as many students as want to learn from us.

While God primarily gains from Salvation being chosen by having closer relationships with more believers, people who teach also gain that benefit ... and much more! To me, it's another indication of God's love for us that He would enable us to benefit more than He does by teaching.

Let me explain why our benefits are greater than from just having closer relationships by sharing my own experiences. While I obviously have a strong desire to be close to and be a help to my family, I am actually closer to some students than to some family members ... without any intent for that difference to occur. Students often pour out their deepest fears, greatest hopes, and biggest problems to me in compelling, candid detail. A family member might, instead, seek to hold back such information from me for a variety of perfectly understandable reasons, including avoiding potential embarrassment. A student is also much more likely to seek counsel from me for how to handle such a daunting problem than a family member who feels motivated to do the opposite, to show that he or she can be effectively independent.

In addition, I receive much joy from seeing students learn something new. I'm sure God is pleased, too, when breakthrough learning is applied to some Godly purpose. In my case, if I can become a more effective teacher, I'll have the opportunity to experience such joy more often in whatever time I devote to teaching. For example, if a student can achieve the same results in one hour that it used to take my students 40 hours in total to achieve, then I can feel that joy 40 times more often. Isn't that great?

If students are so encouraged that they then come back to have me teach them something else, then I have increased joy by hearing more about the benefits they gained from the first learning. In addition, I have the challenge and opportunity for further increasing joy through helping them learn faster and accomplish more during each subsequent time I teach them something new.

When some students apply what they learned in ways that are so original and effective that I learn from them, I have still further increased joy from having contributed a little through God's grace to their accomplishments. In the process, I can also gain insights into how I can work with this student, as well as with others, to have such original and effective contributions occur more frequently.

Finally, I can often learn practical lessons from these students, lessons that I can apply to my nonteaching work. As a result, my breakthrough learning is greatly expanded in ways that could not be easily duplicated in any other way. Why? Well, I can ask a student anything I want about what was done that isn't confidential, and I'll receive full and free disclosure. No one else would do that for me.

As you contemplate these benefits, think a moment about your future. As a believer, you are called to put God first, honoring Him in all ways. Remember, too, that you were created for a purpose, a God-defined and Godly one. In this life, such a purpose will relate to expanding and improving His Kingdom. After this life is over, the Bible tells us that we will be with God for all eternity. While we do not know all of what that means, you probably will not go into any sort of permanent retirement. Instead, we know that God will use us then to help rule His Kingdom:

This is a faithful saying:

For if we died with *Him*,
We shall also live with *Him*.
If we endure,
We shall also reign with *Him*.

— 2 Timothy 2:11-12 (NKJV)

Lesson Twenty-Seven: Improve Your Teaching by Repeating the Steps for Teaching Others

I don't know how you react to that future role in reigning, but I find it mind-boggling. It has been beyond my wildest dreams to be God's servant here on Earth. How could I ever hope to be worthy of reigning with Him? Obviously, God knows the answer, but I don't.

Clearly, our life on Earth must be part of how He is preparing us for our future roles in heaven and on the eventual new Earth. Now, we shouldn't get exaggerated ideas of what such reigning might entail. You and I might be put in charge of inspecting wild goats in a place where no people usually go. However, if God feels that work needs to be done as part of His reign, I'm willing and ready to do it.

Let me raise a possibility in the form of a question: Could there be a relationship between how well we prepare to expand and improve God's Kingdom now and our later role in reigning? That possibility is pretty intriguing to me. Why? I like to learn. I also love to work on expanding and improving God's Kingdom. I greatly enjoy getting to know God better and drawing closer to Him. The possibility seems to connect well to the interests that God has placed in me. Since you are now reading the last lesson in this book after doing quite a bit of learning on your own, chances are good that God made you similarly.

Could it be that Jesus' Parable of the Minas is a reference to how what we do on Earth will affect our future roles for helping Him reign?

> "A certain nobleman went into a far country to receive for himself a kingdom and to return. So he called ten of his servants, delivered to them ten minas, and said to them, 'Do business till I come.'
>
> "But his citizens hated him, and sent a delegation after him, saying, 'We will not have this *man* to reign over us.'

"And so it was that when he returned, having received the kingdom, he then commanded these servants, to whom he had given the money, to be called to him, that he might know how much every man had gained by trading. Then came the first, saying, 'Master, your mina has earned ten minas.'

"And he said to him, 'Well *done*, good servant; because you were faithful in a very little, have authority over ten cities.' And the second came, saying, 'Master, your mina has earned five minas.' Likewise he said to him, 'You also be over five cities.'

"Then another came, saying, 'Master, here is your mina, which I have kept put away in a handkerchief. For I feared you, because you are an austere man. You collect what you did not deposit, and reap what you did not sow.'

"And he said to him, 'Out of your own mouth I will judge you, *you* wicked servant. You knew that I was an austere man, collecting what I did not deposit and reaping what I did not sow. Why then did you not put my money in the bank, that at my coming I might have collected it with interest?'

"And he said to those who stood by, 'Take the mina from him, and give *it* to him who has ten minas.' (But they said to him, 'Master, he has ten minas.') For I say to you, that to everyone who has will be given; and from him who does not have, even what he has will be taken away from him."

— Luke 19:12-26 (NKJV)

While there's no way that we can determine whether the possibility of this intriguing thought is true without God's help, I see no harm in thinking about whatever we learn, whether related to things we do by ourselves or with others ... or what we teach, as possibly being part of God's plan for directing our lives throughout eternity.

Lesson Twenty-Seven: Improve Your Teaching by Repeating the Steps for Teaching Others

Let's think about learning and teaching in a different way. Eternity is a long time. It could get pretty boring unless we have some pretty wonderful things to do. I personally would get tired of playing lots of golf, watching television, or playing video games for all eternity. In fact, I have a hard time thinking of anything to do that wouldn't wear out its attraction. At the same time, when I think about learning or teaching for all eternity, I get excited. I can imagine doing so and being endlessly stimulated. In fact, my mind is instantly filled to overflowing with the possibilities. For instance, are there excellent solutions for composing even greater orchestral music? What would some of the great composers of the past who are now in heaven do with such breakthrough methods? I can hardly wait to hear the sounds!

Now, imagine the alternative to that possibility: No learning and teaching occurs during eternity in heaven. If that's the case, I sure want to do as much of both as I can now. I think that repeating what was just done to teach others is the very best way to do so. As your and my skills increase, we'll be able to teach better ways to accomplish breakthrough learning, as well as teach any higher forms of such learning that God provides ... forms that may well eclipse the most successful excellent solutions of the next few years. Now, isn't that possibility also very exciting? At least from my perspective, it feels like a Godly road of more immense promise than anything else I can do.

So let me raise still another possibility about life on Earth. Could it be that becoming good at breakthrough learning and teaching others to gain such expertise are steps along a pathway for God to give us even greater and more wonderful assignments? While I cannot even begin to imagine what such Earthly work might be, I am certainly excited by the possibility that such an opportunity might be forthcoming.

Here are some reasons to think such might be the case. Since it's challenging and hard work to learn and teach breakthrough learning, our willingness to do so for the purposes of increasing and improving God's Kingdom on Earth certainly shows faithfulness in serving Him. In the course of doing so, we need to rely more on Him than ever before. In doing so, we draw closer to Him. In the course of doing so, we come to know Him better. As we do, His wonderful qualities inspire us to become even more like Jesus. And on it goes.

Let's look at the converse. Let's say that we treat breakthrough learning as the equivalent of a middle-school course we didn't want to take and were happy to forget about as soon as we passed the final. With such an approach, we will not probably do much, if anything, to apply breakthrough learning for increasing and improving God's Kingdom. In that sense, we will be like some of the Pharisees whom Jesus rebuked for talking a good game but not living up to their words. If we are that negligent in using this God-given opportunity, then we are like the unfaithful servants in the parables of the minas and the talents who made no use of what their master had entrusted them with until he returned.

So wouldn't that be the case if we stopped teaching others ways to accomplish breakthrough learning after having done so for the first time? I think so. Do you agree? I hope so.

While you may have your own reasons for thinking, agreeing, and acting in these ways, the important point is to repeat your teaching as often as possible. While I don't know the future, I feel confident that your life here on Earth, as well as in heaven, will be much enhanced if you do. I would hate to see you lose those opportunities. It causes a sharp pain in my heart to even think about the possibility.

If you would like to talk more about continuing your teaching, especially in ways that will increase its fruitfulness, please contact me at the usual e-mail address: donmitchell@fastforward400.com/.

Your Assignments

1. What would you like to improve about your teaching?

2. How might you make such improvements?

Lesson Twenty-Seven: Improve Your Teaching by Repeating the Steps for Teaching Others

3. What would make such improved teaching feel most rewarding to you?

4. How can you increase your focus on finding such opportunities?

5. How can you work more closely with God to direct your future teaching?

Afterword

*Finally, brethren, pray for us,
that the word of the Lord may run swiftly and be glorified,
just as it is with you, and that we may be delivered from
unreasonable and wicked men; for not all have faith.*

*But the Lord is faithful, who will establish you and
guard you from the evil one.
And we have confidence in the Lord concerning you,
both that you do and will do the things we command you.*

*Now may the Lord direct your hearts
into the love of God and into the patience of Christ.*

*But we command you, brethren,
in the name of our Lord Jesus Christ,
that you withdraw from every brother who walks disorderly
and not according to the tradition which he received from us.
For you yourselves know how you ought to follow us,
for we were not disorderly among you;
nor did we eat anyone's bread free of charge,
but worked with labor and toil night and day,
that we might not be a burden to any of you,
not because we do not have authority, but to make ourselves
an example of how you should follow us.
For even when we were with you, we commanded you this:
If anyone will not work, neither shall he eat.
For we hear that there are some who walk among you
in a disorderly manner, not working at all,*

Afterword

> *but are busybodies. Now those who are such we command*
> *and exhort through our Lord Jesus Christ*
> *that they work in quietness and eat their own bread.*
>
> *But as for you, brethren, do not grow weary in doing good.*
> *And if anyone does not obey our word in this epistle,*
> *note that person and do not keep company with him,*
> *that he may be ashamed. Yet do not count* him *as an enemy,*
> *but admonish* him *as a brother.*
>
> — 2 Thessalonians 3:1-15 (NKJV)

In 2 Thessalonians 3:1-15 (NKJV), the Apostle Paul provides us with an appropriate afterword for *Breakthrough Learning*. Bear with me as I build on his excellent points to commission you with the right attitude for applying and teaching breakthrough learning. While I have often mentioned the possibility of applying the breakthrough techniques to lead a more work-free life, my intention in doing so has always been to encourage learners to use the increased time available to live more fruitful lives for God, lives that glorify Him while expanding and improving His Kingdom.

I am sure that you appreciate the opportunity provided by mastering breakthrough learning to spend less time earning a living, and more time living the life that God intended for you. However, our lives are not ours to dispose of as we please. As believers, we belong to God. We are His servants. Some translators point out that the Hebrew word for "servants" is closer to the meaning of "slaves." Ignore the negative connotations you probably have regarding slavery. Following God is more like being with a perfect guide who loves you than an imperfect human slave master who exploits you against your will.

Becoming more adept at breakthrough learning can, in turn, lead you to have a busier life, as you learn and apply more things. In doing so, you'll be a greater blessing to those who need your help. I encourage you to ask God for whom you should seek to be such a greater blessing. As Matthew 25:40 (NKJV) tells us: "Assuredly, I say to you, inasmuch as you did *it* to one of the least of these My brethren, you did *it* to Me." It's one of those wonderful mysteries that we will probably only understand after arriving in heaven, but when we help someone in need, Jesus somehow also receives the benefit. It may be that you should apply some of your new skills to help those who are considered the least of all. Pray about that.

In addition, keep the prior lesson foremost in your mind. Teaching others to become adept at applying and teaching breakthrough learning is probably part of your calling from God, as well. Pray about how He wants you to do so. As you seek His guidance, be aware that God placed on my heart some time ago that the world needs one million tutors of breakthrough methods to best develop His Kingdom. You can read more about what is required in *Help Wanted* (2,000 Percent Living Press, 2011) by me. Ask God if He is calling you to be one of that million. Then, you'll truly become one of a very special million people for Him.

However you choose to apply and teach breakthrough learning, do so to be a blessing to others for increasing and improving God's Kingdom, and you will be blessed in return.

May God bless you, your family, and all you do in the name of Jesus!

Appendix A

Donald Mitchell's Testimony

He will lift you up.

*Humble yourselves
in the sight of the Lord,
and He will lift you up.*

— James 4:10 (NKJV)

Let me share with you how I became a Christian so you will know where I'm coming from with regard to encouraging you to become a Christian and to be fruitful in Godly contributions for creating and implementing breakthrough solutions.

There has been a long commitment to the Lord in our family. For example, I remember my great-grandmother, Edith Foster, reading the Bible every day. As a youngster, my mother regularly took me to Sunday school. It was my least favorite activity; sleeping was much preferred. I did enjoy listening to sermons, but it was frowned on to take youngsters to the adult services where the sermons were given.

If I pretended to be asleep, mom would sometimes let me stay in bed on Sundays. I was pretty good at pretending, and I soon was the biggest backslider in my Sunday school grade. Fortunately, it was an evangelical church so my classmates there were always cooking up schemes to get me to attend again. Because of my high opinion of myself, I would always return if invited to play my clarinet for the congregation.

By the time I turned thirteen, I was pretty full of myself. There wasn't much room for God in there alongside my exaggerated opinion of myself.

One day at home while my family was away for a drive, I felt really sick. By the time they returned, I was delirious. Within an hour, I was in the hospital where I would stay for two weeks as I barely survived a bad case of double pneumonia.

My physician, Dr. Helmsley, was a strong believer in Christ who worried about my soul because my life was in jeopardy. He talked to me about our Heavenly Father, Jesus, and the Holy Spirit twice a day when he stopped by to check on me. These conversations were when I first learned how to become a Christian through being born again. I also came to realize that I couldn't stop sinning on my own. I needed a Savior, Jesus Christ! After I recovered, he took my mom and me to a tent revival meeting.

Having recovered from the illness, I soon pushed God out of my life again. During the next year, I was, instead, very caught up in athletics. When I was in ninth grade, I desperately wanted to make a contribution to our junior high track team, which had a minuscule chance of winning the big meet. Our coach, Mr. Layman, told each of us exactly what had to be accomplished for the team to win. I was determined to do my part. I had to come in first!

But that was not likely to happen. Based on past performances, there were at least two people who could out leap me in the standing broad jump, my main event. To make such a jump, you stand on a slightly raised, forward-tilted board and spring outward as far as you can into a sand-filled pit. After two of the three jumping rounds, I knew it was hopeless. I was in sixth place and four of the competitors' jumps were longer than I had ever gone before. I also didn't like the board we were using.

Remembering that we should call on God when we need help, I thought of praying ... but what I wanted was so trivial in God's terms that I didn't think it was worthy of prayer. So I decided to make God an offer instead: "Dear God, help me win this event, and I'm yours forever." After all, if He came through, any doubts I had about God would be dispelled.

I stepped onto the broad-jump board and felt very calm. I did my routine and took off into the air. Instantly, I felt light as a feather cradled in a large, gentle hand that was lifting me. I was dropped softly at the far end of the pit. I had outleapt everyone and gone more than six inches past my best previous jump. I couldn't believe it. Then I remembered my promise to God, thanked Him, repented my sins, accepted Jesus as my Lord and Savior, and ran off to tell everyone on the team.

Even more remarkable, I was the only person on the team who performed up to the plan. Knowing what had to be done had probably given us performance anxiety, and people underperformed because they didn't believe they could do what the team needed. I also suspect that God wanted to make a point with me that I needed Him.

After a few days, I started to think that perhaps I'd just developed a new broad-jump technique and God didn't have a role at all. God soon dispelled that thought by making sure that my jumps for the rest of my life were much shorter than I had jumped when He lifted me up.

Since then, God has been regularly speaking to me through the Holy Spirit. I have learned to pay attention and to act promptly. When I pursue my own ideas, things don't go so well. When I follow His directions, things work out great. That's my secret to high performance, and I just wanted to share it with you so you could benefit, too. He knows the answers, even when you and I don't ... which is most of the time.

As a management consultant, the Holy Spirit has often filled me with knowledge about what the consequences of one set of actions would be compared to another for my clients. Naturally, I always recommended as the Holy Spirit directed me. Clients often told me that they were impressed by how certain I was of my conclusions and of how persuasive I could be in describing the advantages of whatever recommendations were made. Once again, the explanatory words came from the Holy Spirit, rather than from me.

Unfortunately, I wasn't comfortable in my younger days sharing my faith with clients, and I wrongly gave many people the impression that I was the author of the solutions rather than merely the transmitter.

I wish I had been more faithful in this regard. I apologize to my clients for having missed so many great witnessing opportunities. I didn't always listen as well as I should in making decisions that primarily affected me, but God would always do something to get my attention. Here's an example. I made an investment that I hoped would reduce my taxes in addition to making some money. I didn't have a good feeling from the Holy Spirit at the time, and I shouldn't have invested.

My tax return was later audited by the Internal Revenue Service concerning that investment. It turned out I was in the wrong for the deductions I had taken. Anticipating a big tax bill plus penalties and interest, you can imagine my astonishment when the revised tax return showed me owing no additional money even though I had lost on the audit issues. I knew that result was a gift from God, and I was overwhelmed by His wisdom and power in protecting me. Praise God for His mercy!

I rededicated my life to Jesus in 1995, and I have enjoyed great peace since then. I have also done a lot better in being obedient to the Holy Spirit and to what the Bible tells us to do in all aspects of my life. Many blessings have been mine since then.

After being told by God to start The 400 Year Project (demonstrating how everyone in the world could make improvements 20-times faster and more effectively than normal with no additional resources) in 1995, I continued to receive His instructions. In 2005, for example, God told me to start explaining to people how to live their lives by gaining more joy from what they already have.

In the summer of 2006, I began to see how The 400 Year Project could be brought to a successful conclusion (as I reported in *Adventures of an Optimist*, Mitchell and Company Press, 2007). Realizing that perhaps I had devoted too much of my attention to this one challenge, I began to seek ways to rebalance my life. One of those rebalancing methods was to spend more time communing with God through prayer, Scriptural studies, attending church services and Bible classes, and listening more to the still, small voice within.

For several years I had been enjoying the devotionals sent to me daily over the Internet by evangelist Bill Keller. One of those devotionals pierced me like an arrow that summer. The evangelist reminded his readers that our responsibility as believers is to share our faith with others through our example and sharing the Gospel message from the Bible. Not feeling well equipped to do more than try to be a good example, I began to pray about what else I should be doing.

The next day, my answer came: I was to launch a global contest to locate the most effective ways that souls were being saved and be sure that information was shared widely. This sharing would be a blessing for those who wished to fulfill the Great Commission to spread the Good News of Jesus as commanded in Matthew 28:18-20 (NKJV):

> And Jesus came and spoke to them, saying, "All authority has been given to Me in heaven and on earth. Go therefore and make disciples of all the nations, baptizing them in the name of the Father and of the Son and of the Holy Spirit, teaching them to observe all things that I have commanded you; and lo, I am with you always, *even* to the end of the age."

The contest winners were Jubilee Worship Center in Hobart, Indiana, and Step by Step Ministries in Porter, Indiana. You can read about their experiences to learn amazingly effective ways to help unsaved people choose to accept Salvation in *Witnessing Made Easy: Yes, You Can Make a Difference* (Jubilee Worship Center Step by Step Press, 2010) by Bishop Dale P. Combs, Lisa Combs, Jim Barbarossa, Carla Barbarossa, and me. Six other worthy ideas and practices from the contest for assisting more people to learn about and some of them to be moved by the Holy Spirit to pledge their lives to Jesus are described in a second book, *Ways You Can Witness: How the Lost Are Found* (Salvation Press, 2010) by Cherie Hill, Roger de Brabant, Drew Dickens, Gael Torcise, Wendy Lobos, Herpha Jane Obod, Gisele Umugiraneza, and me.

Let me tell you another interesting thing about my life with Jesus. When my daughter was about a year old, I suffered what resembled a stroke that caused me to start to become paralyzed. As I could feel my face's muscles freezing, I immediately prayed to Jesus to stop the paralysis and He did. I was left with a lot of pain and numbness on the left side of my body and was very weak for over a year.

Part of that pain continued for the next twenty-two years until, on November 8, 2009, I asked two of my pastors during a communion service to pray in the name of Jesus that the remaining pain be removed. During the prayer, the pain started leaving immediately and was totally gone within a half hour. As I felt the pain leaving me, through some power traveling inch by inch down my body, I was overcome with gratitude and fell on my knees in thanks.

That wasn't the only time He recently healed me. Encouraged by that miraculous experience, I came forward again on December 19, 2010, during another communion service to request prayer for relief from the pain in my wrists that was making it difficult for me to write books to serve Him and to do my other work. Knowing that my mother had been plagued with arthritis, I assumed it was a similar onset for me. My pastors were occupied with prayers for other members of the congregation. This time an elder of the church and his wife anointed me with oil and prayed for me. Almost immediately, my whole body shook violently in a way that I couldn't stop. Gradually, the shaking was reduced until it ceased after about half an hour, and my wrist pain was totally gone. It has not returned. I was even more overwhelmed that He had healed me again. Can anyone appreciate all the goodness that God has in store for us?

Let me share yet another miraculous healing (not the last that I've experienced). I have always been troubled with many respiratory and food allergies and sensitivities. In my sixties, these problems had become worse. I finally reached the point where it was difficult to be in the same room with other people due to my reactions to any deodorants and scents they were using. During still another communion service on January 16, 2012, two pastors again prayed for me to be relieved of these problems so that I could be a better witness for Him. Once again, power filled my body. My allergies and sensitivities were gone in a few minutes. Since then, they haven't returned. It has made a huge improvement in my life and in my witnessing.

I have also been saved by God from what I believed to be certain death on twelve occasions, most recently on July 2, 2013. I won't go into all of these events, but I did want you to be aware that He is always touching all aspects of my life in beneficial ways.

While it's up to God to decide if and when He wants to heal us or to protect us from harm, it's certainly reassuring to know that He has the ability and power to do anything He wants.

Glory be to God! Praise Him always! His miracles, grace, and mercy never end. I am so happy and honored to be His servant and witness to you.

Appendix B

Summary of The 400 Year Project

*Therefore we also pray always for you
that our God would count you worthy of this calling,
and fulfill all the good pleasure of His goodness
and the work of faith with power,
that the name of our Lord Jesus Christ
may be glorified in you, and you in Him,
according to the grace of our God
and the Lord Jesus Christ.*

— 2 Thessalonians 1:11-12 (NKJV)

One morning during the summer of 1995 at around 3:45 a.m., I felt a warm presence fill the bedroom. In response, my body temperature seemed to rise and I felt deliriously happy. A voice that I didn't recognize filled my mind and told me in tones that were more resonant and powerful than James Earl Jones on his best day that I should hold a meeting for all of my management consulting clients to celebrate and share their greatest accomplishments on that year's autumnal equinox. At the end of the meeting, I should announce that I would be starting a 20-year project to find ways for the whole world to make 400 years of normal progress in only 20 years, beginning in 2015 and finishing in 2035. For the next few weeks, I could think of little else.

Appendix B: Summary of The 400 Year Project

What had happened? I prayed over the experience quite a bit and concluded that God had sent me a message. Why me? I have no idea. Maybe He couldn't find anyone else crazy enough to take on such an impossible task. I certainly felt that only God would know how to do it.

Why that time frame? I don't know, but it later occurred to me that the 2,000th anniversary of Jesus' crucifixion and resurrection would occur during 2015–2035. Perhaps that was an important connection. Since then, I've come to appreciate that 20 is a spiritually important number to God: Notice that the dimensions of the Holy of Holies in the Temple were measured in terms of 20 cubits. But who knows, except God?

How would I pursue this project? I had no idea, not even a clue. All I knew was that I was supposed to make this announcement at the autumnal equinox.

I quickly organized the meeting. Clients graciously agreed to fly in to share their triumphs and lessons with one another. Not knowing how anyone else would take the announcement of the new project, I decided to keep it to myself. I also had the impression that I should keep the project private until the announcement. Otherwise, why make the announcement then rather than sooner?

The event went much better than I could have hoped, especially since I was not sure what to say during the unexpected announcement. Almost all listeners were encouraging, and many volunteered to help with the project.

A key early focus was to engage in writing a book that Peter Drucker, the founder of the management discipline, had encouraged Carol Coles and me to write encapsulating a problem-solving method that we had been using for many years. We were fortunate to gain the assistance of Robert Metz, a veteran author and journalist, as a coauthor to lead us through the publication twists and turns. That book was *The 2,000 Percent Solution*, still the most widely read publication produced by The 400 Year Project.

Having experienced a warm reception for this book, I was delighted when the Holy Spirit kept providing concepts, processes, or the actual words for many future books, of which twenty more have been completed with the publication of this new book, *Breakthrough Learning*. Through these books, readers and my students have created their own breakthroughs by employing The 400 Year Project's methods. I'm aware of successful demonstration projects that have been conducted so far in over 60 countries. There are probably more such successes that I'm unaware of. What a blessing! Praise God!

I have also had the pleasure of conducting several global contests, building experience to supplement the concepts first articulated in *The Ultimate Competitive Advantage* about this way of making rapid advances.

I also established a learning organization, The Billionaire Entrepreneurs' Master Mind, to advance how complementary 2,000 percent solutions could be most effectively developed and combined. I continue to be delighted by the lessons developed by that group, which have richly informed *Business Basics* and the three books in the recently completed Advanced Business series.

Today, The 400 Year Project is ready for prime time. The books, experiences, and networks of breakthrough problem solvers provide a sound foundation for expanding and transforming God's Kingdom in every possible dimension between now and 2035 by far more than 20 times. I am truly delighted that you will be part of creating such remarkable transformations.

May God bless you, your family, and all you do in the name of Jesus!